D1247205

Imaging of the Chest
A Teaching File

Imaging of the Chest
A Teaching File

Patricia J. Mergo, M.D.

Associate Professor
Division of Thoracic and Body Imaging
Director of Computed Tomography and Thoracic Imaging
Department of Radiology
University of Florida College of Medicine
Gainesville, Florida

LIPPINCOTT WILLIAMS & WILKINS
A **Wolters Kluwer** Company

Philadelphia · Baltimore · New York · London
Buenos Aires · Hong Kong · Sydney · Tokyo

Acquisitions Editor: Joyce-Rachel John
Developmental Editor: Marc Bendian
Production Editor: Rosemary Palumbo
Manufacturing Manager: Tim Reynolds
Cover Designer: Mark Lerner
Compositor: Maryland Composition Company, Inc.
Printer: Maple Press

Printed in the USA

Library of Congress Cataloging-in-Publication Data

Mergo, Patricia J.
    Imaging of the chest : a teaching file / Patricia J. Mergo.
      p. ; cm.
    Includes bibliographical references and index.
    ISBN 0-683-30473-9
      1. Chest–Radiography. 2. Chest–Diseases–Case studies. I. Title.
    [DNLM: 1. Thoracic Diseases–radiography. 2. Diagnostic Imaging–methods. WF 975
M559i 2002]
    RC941 .M367 2002
    617.5'407572–dc21   2001033878

10 9 8 7 6 5 4 3 2 1

To my family—
My husband, Brian L. Kiel; my children, Casey Alexander Kiel and Kaitlyn Nicole Kiel;
and my parents, Nicholas J. and Margaret W. Mergo.

CONTENTS

CONTRIBUTING AUTHORS

Alfredo L. Arraut, M.D. *Resident, Department of Radiology, University of Texas Southwestern Medical Center, Dallas, Texas*

Thomas Dunphy, M.D. *Chief Resident, Department of Radiology, University of Florida College of Medicine, Gainesville, Florida*

Runi A. Foster, M.D. *Clinical Assistant Professor, Department of Medicine, University of Florida College of Medicine; and Division of Pulmonary Medicine, Department of Medicine, Shands Hospital, Gainesville, Florida*

Megan C. Hodge, M.D. *Resident, Department of Radiology, University of Florida College of Medicine and Shands Hospital, Gainesville, Florida*

Michael J. Jurgens, M.D. *Resident, Department of Radiology, University of Florida College of Medicine, Gainesville, Florida*

Tammy Edwards Kitchens, M.D. *Resident, Department of Radiology, University of Florida College of Medicine, Gainesville, Florida*

Patricia J. Mergo, M.D. *Associate Professor, Division of Thoracic and Body Imaging, Director of Computed Tomography and Thoracic Imaging, Department of Radiology, University of Florida College of Medicine, Gainesville, Florida*

Allison E. Tonkin, M.D. *Resident, Department of Radiology, University of Florida College of Medicine, Gainesville, Florida*

PUBLISHER'S FOREWORD

Teaching Files are one of the hallmarks of education in radiology. There has long been a need for a comprehensive series of books, using the Teaching File format, that would provide the kind of personal consultation with the experts normally found only in the setting of a teaching hospital. Lippincott Williams & Wilkins is proud to have created such a series; our goal is to provide the resident and practicing radiologist with a useful resource that answers this need.

Actual cases have been culled from extensive teaching files in major medical centers. The discussions presented mimic those performed on a daily basis between residents and faculty members in all radiology departments.

The format of this series is designed so that each case can be studied as an unknown, if desired. A consistent format is used to present each case. A brief clinical history is given, followed by several images. Then, relevant findings, differential diagnosis, and final diagnosis are given, followed by a discussion of the case. The authors thereby guide the reader through the interpretation of each case.

We hope that this series will become a valuable and trusted teaching tool for radiologists at any stage of training or practice, and that it will also be a benefit to clinicians whose patients undergo these imaging studies.

The Publisher

PREFACE

This teaching file textbook on imaging of the chest consists of 150 cases of diseases of the thorax (with approximately 390 images), arranged in categories according to patterns of their radiographic appearance. Each case is presented as an unknown entity with a pertinent history given, followed by the radiographic findings, the diagnosis, and a discussion of the disease process, and, when pertinent, a differential diagnosis. The radiographic findings and pattern of disease are emphasized, including the plain chest radiography findings and, in many cases the CT and MR imaging findings.

The goal of this text is to provide practicing radiologists and radiology residents preparing for board examinations with a comprehensive book that illustrates the radiographic findings of pertinent thoracic diseases, discusses the key findings, and offers a concise differential diagnosis. The inclusion of clinical presentations and key clinical information provides the clinician with an overview of radiographic presentations of pulmonary diseases, and fosters the development of a pattern recognition approach to chest radiography and cross-sectional imaging.

Our approach covers the gamut of the most common types of disease encountered in the thorax, and not only lists the diseases, but shows prime examples of the entities discussed. It is this approach which I hope the reader will find most useful and unique, whether he or she is a fourth-year resident in radiology preparing for the boards, or a pulmonologist who wants to further their understanding of thoracic imaging. The goal in creating this book was not to create a book of lists of differential diagnoses, but to take common lists of differential diagnoses and build upon them, showing examples of radiographic findings that would help the reader create a pattern recognition approach to decipher these lists and narrow in on the proper diagnosis. This is not possible in every instance, but serves as an overall philosophy for the style of this textbook.

Patricia J. Mergo, M.D.

ACKNOWLEDGMENTS

Many individuals helped in the preparation of this book. First, I would like to acknowledge my family, who have supported me throughout my career as well as throughout the preparation of this textbook. I thank my husband Brian, my parents, Nick and Peggy Mergo, and Genie, Sylvia, and Nick for their love and support. I thank my two-year-old son, Casey Alexander, for his uncanny ability to provide me with comic relief and perspective, and my four-week-old daughter, Kaitlyn Nicole, for snoozing through her entire first month of life, enabling me to finish the manuscript.

John Bisigni, Marc Gualtieri, and Beth Bethea, as undergraduate students, helped me compile the cases for this book over many years. Without their assistance in the organization of this material, this task would have been nearly insurmountable.

I would like to thank the members of the Division of Pulmonary Medicine at the University of Florida College of Medicine, including Eloise Harman, Runi Foster, Ricardo Gonzalez-Rothi, Michael Cicale, Michael Jantz, Marc Brantly, Gene Ryerson, Maher Baz, Rich Berry, Ed Block, and Jay Block, for their input on many of the cases presented in this book.

My colleagues and former colleagues, Patricia L. Abbitt, Pablo R. Ros, Gladys M. Torres, and Sharon S. Burton provided guidance, hard work, dedication, and a nurturing environment which aided in the completion of the manuscript. Linda Funk-Waters helped with the manuscript preparation.

ABBREVIATIONS AND ACRONYMS

AIDS	acquired immunodeficiency syndrome
AILD	angioimmunoblastic lymphadenopathy
ANCA	antineutrophil cytoplasmic antibodies
AP	anteroposterior
ARDS	adult respiratory distress syndrome
BAC	bronchioloalveolar carcinoma
BHL	bilateral hilar lymphadenopathy
BOOP	bronchiolitis obliterans with organizing pneumonia
CECT	contrast-enhanced computed tomography
CIP	chronic interstitial pneumonitis
CLL	chronic lymphocytic leukemia
CMV	cytomegalovirus
COPD	chronic obstructive pulmonary disease
CREST	calcinosis, Raynaud's syndrome, esophageal dysmotility, sclerodactyly, and telangiectasis
CT	computed tomography
DIP	desquamative interstitial pneumonia
DVT	deep venous thrombosis
EG	eosinophilic granuloma
GBM	glomerular basement membrane
HIV	human immunodeficiency virus
HRCT	high-resolution computed tomography
INH	isonicotinic acid hydrazide
IPF	idiopathic pulmonary fibrosis
KTWS	Klippel-Trenaunay-Weber syndrome
LAM	lymphangioleiomyomatosis
LDH	lactate dehydrogenase
MAI	*Mycobacterium avium-intracellulare*
MRI	magnetic resonance imaging
NF	neurofibromatosis
PA	posteroanterior
PAP	pulmonary alveolar proteinosis
PAWP	pulmonary artery wedge pressures
PCP	*Pneumocystis carinii* pneumonia
PE	pulmonary embolism
PMF	progressive massive fibrosis
PNET	primitive neuroectodermal tumor
PPD	purified protein derivative of tuberculin
RML	right middle lobe
RMLS	right middle lobe syndrome
RSV	respiratory syncytial virus
SCUBA	self contained underwater breathing apparatus
SIADH	syndrome of inappropriate secretion of antidiuretic hormone
SLE	systemic lupus erythematosus
SVC	superior vena cava
TB	tuberculosis
TE	tracheoesophageal
TIPS	transjugular intrahepatic portosystemic shunt
UIP	usual interstitial pneumonia
VATER complex	vertebral, anal, cardiac, tracheoesophageal, and renal anomalies
VSD	ventricular septal defect

CHAPTER 1

PATTERNS OF LOBAR COLLAPSE

PATRICIA J. MERGO

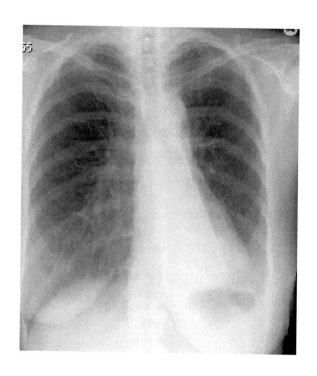

CASE 1

History: A 35-year-old woman with a history of smoking one pack of cigarettes per day for 15 years presents with progressive right upper quadrant pain, and right-sided chest pain.

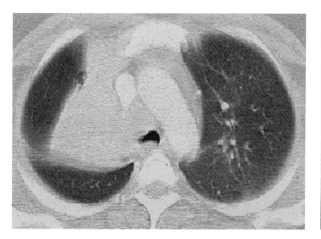

Figure 1A

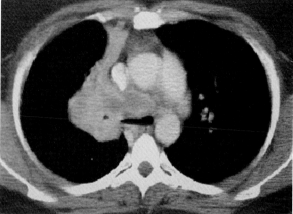

Figure 1B

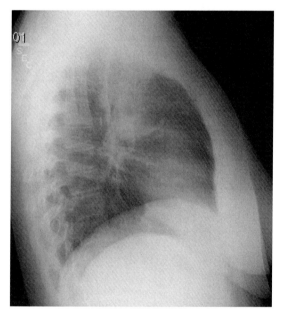

Figure 1C

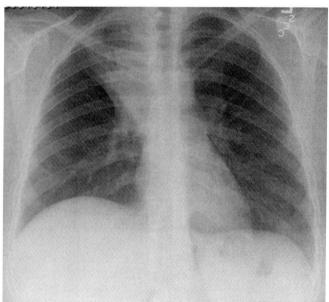

Figure 1D

Findings: Multiple bilateral lung nodules were noted, right greater than left, with a large focal right suprahilar mass, collapse of the right upper lobe, superior bowing of the minor fissure, and a large pretracheal lymph node with subcarinal lymphadenopathy.

Diagnosis: Poorly differentiated non–small cell carcinoma of the lung, with right upper lobe collapse and S sign of Golden.

Discussion: The right upper lobe collapses superiorly and medially with increased opacity evident in the right upper zone, which is delineated inferiorly by the horizontal fissure. With right upper lobe collapse, there is elevation of the minor fissure, shift of the trachea to the right, and elevation of the right hilum. Density or thickening along the right paratracheal region may be seen. Right upper lobe collapse is less visible on the lateral film because the upper zone is often partly obscured by the overlying soft tissues, shoulders, and upper arms. Endobronchial tumor, tumor encasement of a bronchus, mucous plugging, and scarring from old granulomatous disease are common causes of right upper lobe collapse.

The S sign of Golden is demonstrated in this case and is created by an obstructing central mass that produces a convexity along the interface of the collapsed upper lobe and the hyperinflated middle lobe. The convexity of the mass in continuity with the concavity of the more distal portion of the right upper lobe–RML interface produces the characteristic S shape. The S sign of Golden can be considered a secondary sign of malignancy.

Collapse of the left upper lobe has a similar appearance, but with left upper lobe collapse there is no sharp line of demarcation as is seen on the right, which is attributable to the presence of the horizontal fissure on the right. The left upper lobe collapses anteriorly, causing a hazy opacity over the left hemithorax, which is more dense toward the lung apex. The lower lobe becomes hyperexpanded behind the collapsed left upper lobe, and the aortic knob is clearly visualized.

CASE 2

History: A 36-year-old woman reported feeling ill for approximately 2 months with a poor appetite, a productive cough and a 10-pound weight loss. She found that if she lay on her right side at night that she choked secondary to the production of thick purulent sputum. She had occasional sharp mid-sternal chest pain and a history of smoking one pack of cigarettes per day for 25 years. Fiberoptic bronchoscopy showed no endobronchial lesion. Biopsies and washings were negative for tumor.

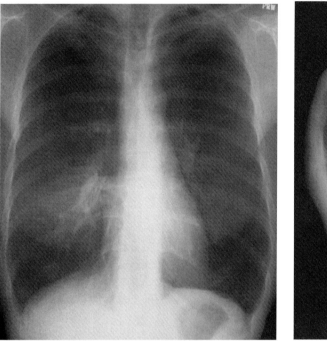

Figure 2A

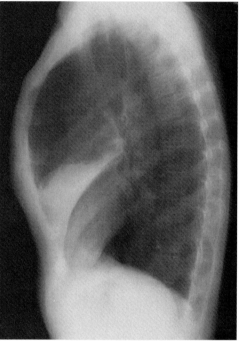

Figure 2B

Findings: PA and lateral chest radiographs showed a wedge-shaped opacity overlying the heart border (*B*) and obscuring the right heart border (*A*).

Diagnosis: Right middle lobe syndrome (RMLS).

Discussion: This patient's pattern of recurrent infection of the RML is consistent with a diagnosis of RMLS. RMLS is a pattern of recurrent or chronic atelectasis of the RML that results in recurrent lobar pneumonia. There are two major theories regarding the underlying pathophysiology.

The first theory suggests that central obstruction is the cause of the recurrent atelectasis. The RML bronchus has the smallest diameter of all the lobar bronchi. It is a long structure and has relatively little cartilage in its wall. The RML bronchus is surrounded by lymph nodes that become enlarged after pneumonia or tuberculosis. These nodes may compress the bronchus, causing atelectasis and promoting infection.

A newer theory suggests that RMLS is caused by a relative lack of collateral ventilation. Collateral ventilation through the pores of Kohn may maintain aeration of alveoli when airways are obstructed by secretions. This prevents reabsorption of gas in the distal alveoli and, by keeping air in the alveoli, allows the cough mechanism to remove secretions from the airway. Collateral ventilation does not occur across lobar boundaries; hence, the two segments that make up the RML can only provide collateral ventilation for the other. In contrast, the segments that make up the other lobes are in contact with and can receive collateral ventilation from at least two other segments.

Right middle lobe syndrome manifests on imaging studies as recurrent or chronic RML consolidation or atelectasis. On anterior chest films, atelectasis of the RML may be difficult to detect. An opacity is not always visible, and it is more useful to look for a loss of the silhouette of the right heart border. The opacity is readily seen on lateral films and has a concave lower border. This distinguishes it from fluid in the minor fissure, which presents with a convex lower margin. On CT, RML atelectasis appears as a triangular density adjoining the mediastinum. This opacity may look similar to a loculated collection in the pleural space by the presence of the RML bronchus entering posteromedially.

CASE 3

History: A 45-year-old female nonsmoker with progressive shortness of breath, inspiratory wheezing and squeaking, pleuritic chest pain on deep inspiration, nonproductive cough, and left lower lobe endobronchial lesion on bronchoscopy.

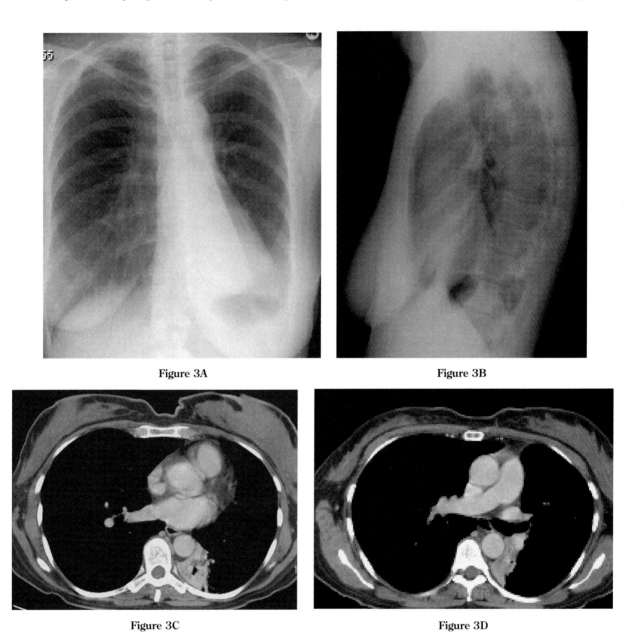

Figure 3A

Figure 3B

Figure 3C

Figure 3D

Findings: PA and lateral chest radiographs showed increased opacity in the left retrocardiac region with volume loss in the left hemithorax. CT of the chest showed collapse of the left lobe of the lung with no definite endobronchial lesions.

Diagnosis: Carcinoid tumor.

Discussion: The left lower lobe, like the right lower lobe, collapses medially and posteriorly toward the mediastinum. The left hilum is displaced inferiorly, and there also may be elevation of the left hemidiaphragm, shift of the heart to the left, and compensatory hyperinflation of the left upper lobe. Classically, a triangular opacity may be seen behind the heart, giving the cardiac silhouette an unusually straight lateral border. The left hemidiaphragm also may be obscured by the collapsed lobe.

A patient with a collapsed lung on imaging should undergo follow-up bronchoscopy to evaluate the cause of the collapse for definitive diagnosis and treatment. Endobronchial neoplasms may include carcinoid tumors (90% of tumors) and bronchial gland tumors such as adenoid cystic carcinoma (8%) and mucoepidermoid carcinoma (2%). Other endobronchial obstructing lesions include pedunculated hamartomas, foreign bodies, and mucous plugs.

CASE 4

History: An 81-year-old woman was undergoing a preoperative routine workup prior to glaucoma surgery. A preoperative chest radiograph was obtained as part of the evaluation.

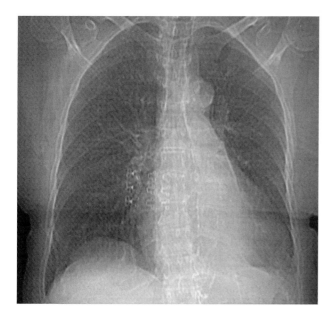

Figure 4A

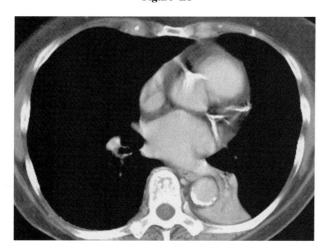

Figure 4B

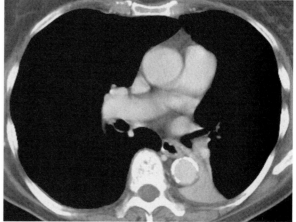

Figure 4C

Findings: A scout image from a CT examination showed a triangular opacity behind the heart border on the frontal view. The cardiac silhouette was distinct from the atelectatic lower lobe. Two images from a contrast-enhanced CT of the chest showed collapse of the lower lobe posteriorly. No endobronchial lesion was seen, and the left upper lobe was compensatorily hyperexpanded.

Diagnosis: Left lower lobe collapse.

Discussion: The classic triangular opacity seen through the cardiac silhouette of left lower lobe collapse is well demonstrated in this case, giving the cardiac silhouette an unusually straight lateral border. This case also demonstrates the partial obscuration of the left hemidiaphragm, where the collapsed portion of lung abuts the hemidiaphragm posteriorly.

This patient underwent bronchoscopic evaluation after CT was performed and was found to have no endobronchial lesion. Her airways were diffusely edematous and inflamed, and thick and purulent secretions were noted in both the right and left bronchi and were removed from the left lower lobe. She had no further documented episodes of collapse after bronchoscopy was performed.

CASE 5

History: A 67-year-old woman with a long history of recurrent episodes of cough and occasional chest pain.

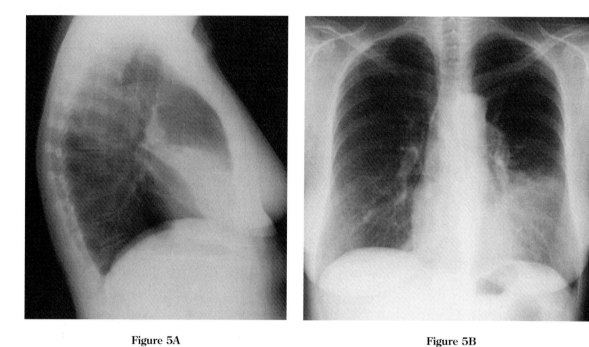

Figure 5A   Figure 5B

Findings: PA and lateral radiographs of the chest demonstrated obliteration of the left heart border (PA film), with increased opacity in the left lung base adjacent to the cardiac silhouette. The lateral film demonstrated a wedge-shaped opacity noted anteriorly with volume loss evident in the lingula. Careful examination of the chest x-ray demonstrated calcified lymph nodes within both hilar regions.

Diagnosis: Recurrent left lingular atelectasis related to obstruction from a broncholith.

Discussion: Lingular atelectasis causes obliteration of the left heart border with an anterior wedge-shaped opacity overlying the heart evident on the lateral film and associated volume loss.

Recurrent episodes of atelectasis should be further evaluated for underlying endobronchial abnormalities. At bronchoscopy, a broncholith was seen in the left lingular bronchus as the cause of obstruction.

SUGGESTED READING

Ashizawa K, Hayashi K, Aso N, et al. Lobar atelectasis: diagnostic pitfalls on chest radiography. *Br J Radiol* 2001;74:89–97.

Liu S, Ko S, Chen W. Bronchial carcinoid tumor presenting with complete lobar collapse and unilateral lung emphysema. *Clin Imaging* 2000;24:159–161.

Nimkin K, Kleinman PK, Zwerdling RG, et al. Localized pneumothorax with lobar collapse and diffuse obstructive airway disease. *Pediatr Radiol* 1995;25:449–451.

Onitsuka H, Tsukuda M, Araki A, et al. Differentiation of central lung tumor from postobstructive lobar collapse by rapid sequence computed tomography. *J Thorac Imaging* 1991;6:28–31.

Proto AV, Tocino I. Radiographic manifestations of lobar collapse. *Semin Roentgenol* 1980;15:117–173.

Su WJ, Lee PY, Perng RP. Chest roentgenographic guidelines in the selection of patients for fiberoptic bronchoscopy. *Chest* 1993;103:1198–1201.

Woodring JH, Reed JC. Types and mechanisms of pulmonary atelectasis. *J Thorac Imaging* 1996;11:92–108.

CHAPTER 2

AIRSPACE DISEASE

ALFREDO L. ARRAUT
PATRICIA J. MERGO

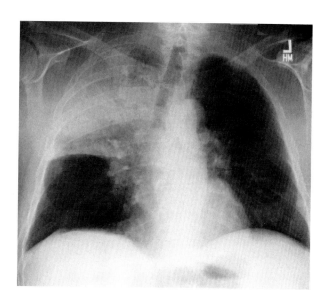

CASE 6

History: A 60-year-old white man with a history of COPD, ischemic cardiomyopathy, congestive heart failure, gastroesophageal reflux, and gastritis. He presented with a 4-day history of suddenly worsening pleuritic chest pain. He also complained of fever, rigors, and cough productive of yellow sputum. He was admitted four times for bacterial pneumonia in the preceding 2 years.

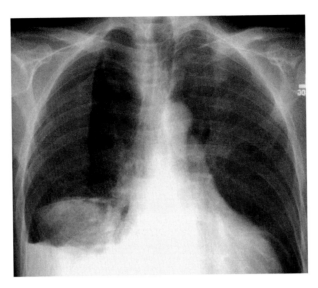

Figure 6

Findings: A single frontal radiographic view of the chest showed complete consolidation of the right middle lobe and a large hydropneumothorax on the right side.

Differential Diagnosis: Bacterial, fungal, and mycobacterial infections can give this appearance. BAC is also a consideration. Pleural fluid was removed and found to be exudative, with a white blood cell count of 23,000 cells/mm^3 and protein of 3.0 g/dL. Pleural fluid and sputum cultures yielded no organisms. The patient was treated with antibiotics and subsequently improved.

Diagnosis: Bacterial lobar pneumonia.

Discussion: There are four basic radiographic patterns of infective pneumonia: bronchopneumonia and spherical, interstitial, and lobar pneumonia. In bronchopneumonia, there is multifocal filling of the large airways with inflammatory exudate that spreads to the surrounding acini, giving a nodular pattern of patchy consolidation. It can be caused by TB or bacterial abscesses. Because the airways are filled, there are no air bronchograms. Obstruction of the bronchi leads to loss of volume.

Spherical or round pneumonia is most frequently seen in children. It presents as an ill-defined round area of consolidation with or without air bronchograms. Interstitial pneumonia presents as widespread peribronchial thickening and ill-defined reticulonodular shadowing. It is commonly caused by viral or *Mycoplasma* pneumonia.

Community-acquired pneumonias most often present as lobar pneumonia. The inflammatory exudate begins by filling the distal air spaces. It may spread across segmental boundaries through the pores of Kohn, resulting in homogenous consolidation bound by fissures. Air bronchograms may be seen within the area of consolidation. The airways are not affected, and no loss of volume is seen. Postobstructive pneumonia should be considered in cases of lobar pneumonia, especially if there are recurrent pneumonias of the same lobe.

CASE 7

History: A 25-year-old black man presented to the emergency room with a 3-day history of productive cough, pleuritic chest pain, and fevers.

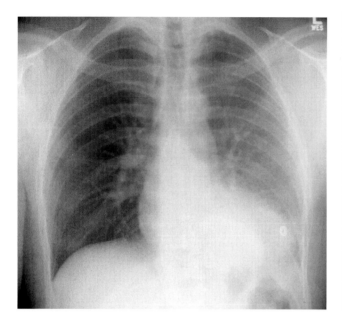

Figure 7A

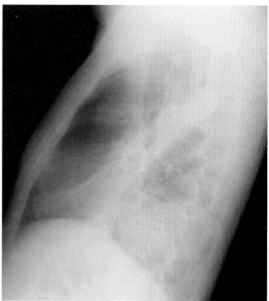

Figure 7B

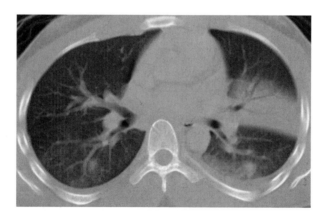

Figure 7C

Findings: On chest x-ray, there was a left lower lobe opacity and left-sided pleural effusion. There was also fluid in the major fissure. CT showed a dense consolidation with air bronchograms in the posterior portion of the left upper lobe and left lower lobe, as well as patchy consolidation of the right lower lobe.

Differential Diagnosis: This is most likely an infectious pneumonia of bacterial, fungal, or mycobacterial etiology. Blood cultures grew out *Pneumococcus*.

Diagnosis: Pneumococcal pneumonia.

Discussion: This patient had a *Streptococcus pneumoniae* pneumonia involving the left upper and lower lobe, with possible involvement of the right lower lobe. *S. pneumoniae* is a gram-positive coccus that grows in pairs or chains. It causes a zone of alpha hemolysis when grown on blood agar and is distinguished by its high sensitivity to optochin. There are about 90 serotypes of pneumococcus, although 85% of infections in humans are caused by 1 of the 23 serotypes that are included in the commercially available vaccine.

Pneumococcus is reported to be the number one cause of community-acquired bacterial pneumonia, as well as the number one etiology of pneumonias requiring hospitalization. It can affect patients of any age, although the elderly, asplenic patients, multiple myeloma patients, alcoholics, and patients with congestive heart failure or influenza are at higher risk. Winter and early spring are the peak seasons for infection. The bacteria usually colonize the oropharynx before causing pneumonia, and it is estimated that 20% to 40% of the general population is colonized.

Symptoms of pneumococcal pneumonia include chills, fevers, cough productive of red or rusty sputum, and pleuritic chest pain. White blood cell counts often exceed 15,000 cells/mm^3, and the proportion of neutrophils is greater than 80%. Intravenous beta-lactam antibiotic or a combination of ampicillin, sulbactam, and a macrolide are the recommended regimens for empiric treatment of inpatients with suspected pneumococcal pneumonia. With proper treatment, the patient's clinical condition improves within 48 hours, and complete resolution occurs within 2 weeks. There has been growing concern over the increased incidence of beta-lactam–resistant pneumococcus, which is especially common in children.

The classic radiographic appearance is that of a homogenous, nonsegmental consolidation abutting a pleural margin, with an irregular edge of advancing alveolar involvement. Air bronchograms may be present. More recent studies suggest that patchy bronchopneumonic consolidation may be a more common pattern of appearance. This pattern is more widespread, but does not often involve more than one lobe. Irregular linear interstitial and mixed interstitial/bronchopulmonary patterns also have been reported. Underlying conditions do not seem to affect the presenting pattern. Parapneumonic effusions are commonly seen on CT and can progress to empyema.

CASE 8

History: A 63-year-old white woman was admitted to the hospital with refractory acute myelogenous leukemia. The patient had persistent fevers throughout her hospitalization. Serial pan cultures failed to reveal an organism. She also complained of fatigue, weakness, and a nonproductive cough.

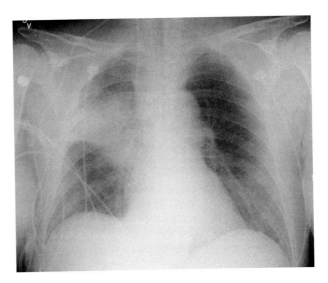

Figure 8

Findings: A single frontal radiographic view of the chest demonstrated a rounded opacity in the upper lobe of the right lung, consistent with pneumonia. The opacity is located above the fissure with downward displacement of the fissure.

Diagnosis: Right upper lobe pneumonia.

Discussion: There are four basic radiographic patterns of infective pneumonia: bronchopneumonia and round, interstitial, and lobar pneumonia. In bronchopneumonia, there is multifocal filling of the large airways with inflammatory exudate that spreads to the surrounding acini, giving a nodular pattern of patchy consolidation. It can be caused by TB or bacterial abscesses. Because the airways are filled, there are no air bronchograms. Obstruction of the bronchi leads to loss of volume.

Round or spherical pneumonia is most frequently seen in children. It presents as an ill-defined round area of consolidation with or without air bronchograms. Interstitial pneumonia presents as widespread peribronchial thickening and ill-defined reticulonodular shadowing. It is commonly caused by viral or *Mycoplasma* pneumonia.

Community-acquired pneumonias most often present as lobar pneumonia. The inflammatory exudate begins by filling the distal air spaces, spreading across segmental boundaries through the pores of Kohn, resulting in homogenous consolidation bound by fissures, which may exhibit air bronchograms. The airways are not affected, and no loss of volume is seen. Postobstructive pneumonia should be considered in cases of lobar pneumonia, especially if there are recurrent pneumonias of the same lobe.

CASE 9

History: A 68-year-old white man with chronic lymphocytic leukemia, whose white blood cell count had been increasing steadily over the preceding 3 months presented to the clinic complaining of worsening constitutional symptoms, including fatigue, shortness of breath, cold sweats, and splenic pain.

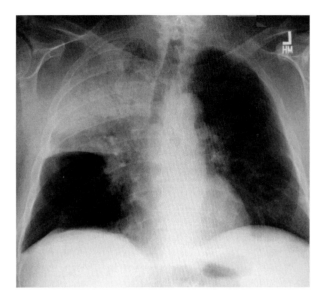

Figure 9A

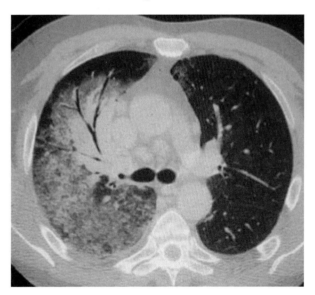

Figure 9B

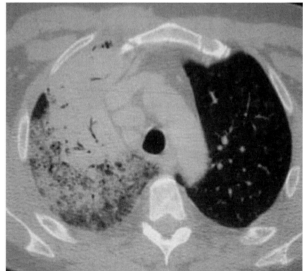

Figure 9C

Findings: A single frontal view of the chest and selected images from CT of the chest without contrast showed right upper lobe consolidation with air bronchograms. No obstructive mass was seen. The superior segment of the right lower lobe was also involved. There was right paratracheal, left hilar, and precarinal adenopathy.

Differential Diagnosis: Infectious pneumonia from bacterial causes is most common, but because of the patient's immunocompromised status, other unusual infections must be considered. These include viral, mycobacterial, fungal, and PCP.

Diagnosis: Right upper lobe adenovirus pneumonia.

Discussion: Community-acquired respiratory viral infections are an important problem in patients with cancer. Eighteen percent of adult leukemia patients hospitalized for an acute respiratory illness have a community-acquired viral infection. Of these, most are caused by RSV, influenza, or picornaviruses. Adenovirus infection is less common but clinically significant. As many as 63% of community-acquired respiratory viral infections are complicated by pneumonia, and the associated mortality rate is 47%. Adenovirus is different from the other pathogens in several ways. It is a DNA virus, whereas the others are based on RNA. Illness may be caused by exogenous infection or by reactivation of an endogenous infection, although existing evidence suggests that the former is responsible for most clinically significant cases. Unlike the other viruses, pneumonias in leukemia patients caused by adenovirus are not preceded by upper respiratory infection.

The diagnosis of adenovirus pneumonia is complicated by the fact that there are more than 47 serotypes. The incidence of these serotypes in sick immunocompromised patients is clustered by the patient's age and nature of immunosuppression. Diagnosis is further complicated by the fact that the clinical and histopathologic appearance is very similar to RSV infection. The most common radiographic appearance is bilateral patchy consolidation, but, as in this patient, it can appear as consolidation confined predominantly to one lobe. In these cases, it is important to differentiate this entity from a bacterial pneumonia. Other prominent radiographic findings include bronchial wall thickening and peribronchial shadowing. As many as a third of patients will have a small pleural effusion. Children are prone to lobar collapse, most commonly of the right upper or left lower lobes. Many patients recover without sequelae, but childhood infection is correlated with increased incidence of chronic problems such as bronchiectasis and obliterative bronchiolitis.

CASE 10

History: A 40-year-old African-American man who was involved in a house fire. He sustained 12% total body surface area burns and inhalation injuries. He was intubated at the scene. During his hospitalization, he developed pulmonary infiltrates on chest radiographs.

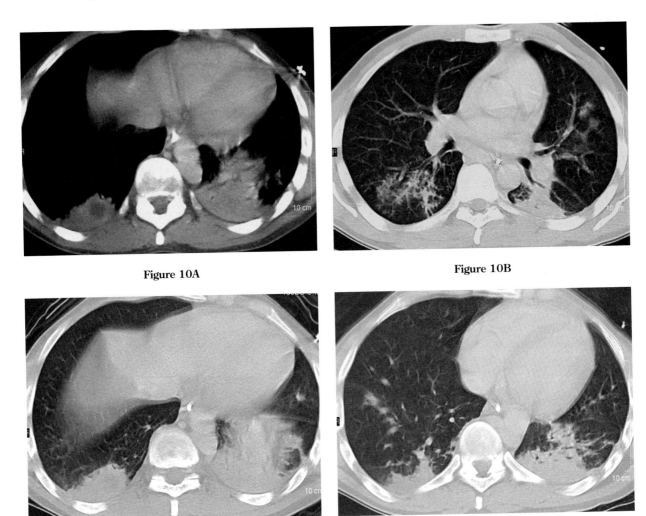

Figure 10A

Figure 10B

Figure 10C

Figure 10D

Findings: CT demonstrated bilateral basilar consolidation and a 3-cm pleural-based cavitary lesion in the right lower lobe. There was also bilateral peribronchial thickening and inflammatory changes. There was acinar filling in the right lower lobe, giving a tree-and-bud appearance (*B*).

Differential Diagnosis: The pattern of necrotizing consolidation is consistent with gram-negative or anaerobic pneumonia. *Staphylococcus aureus, Actinomyces,* and fungal pneumonias also should be included in the differential diagnosis. Sputum cultures grew out *Klebsiella pneumoniae.*

Diagnosis: *Klebsiella* pneumonia.

Discussion: Gram-negative bacteria are an important group of pulmonary pathogens that are capable of causing both nosocomial and community-acquired pneumonia. Gram-negative bacteria are the most common pathogens in hospital-acquired pneumonia. In the community setting, gram-negative infections are most commonly seen in chronic alcoholics. Chronic alcoholism contributes to the disease process by decreasing the host defense mechanisms. It causes decreased ciliary function and surfactant production, and also interferes with neutrophil migration and macrophage activity. *Klebsiella* pneumonia, in particular, is seen almost exclusively in alcoholics.

Klebsiella pneumoniae causes a lobar pneumonia that presents with high fevers and other systemic symptoms. Chest radiographs show a quickly spreading consolidation with a sharp margin. Some series report an association with lobar expansion on plain films, but this does not appear to be a common occurrence. In contrast to pneumococcal pneumonia, *Klebsiella* pneumonia is associated with a tendency to cavitate or form chronic abscesses. In general, consolidation with cavitation strongly suggests gram-negative or anaerobic infection. *S. aureus* and fungal pneumonias are also considerations. Pulmonary gangrene, a term denoting massive necrosis of lung parenchyma, is a rare complication of *Klebsiella* infection.

On CT, *Klebsiella* pneumonia appears as a lobar consolidation with a mix of enhancing areas and poorly demarcated areas of hypoattenuation containing small cavities. The poorly enhancing areas are thought to be regions of necrosis with early cavitation.

Klebsiella pneumonia is a particularly severe disease in alcoholic patients, whose mortality rate may range from 50% to 60%. Bacteremia in these patients is correlated with a poor prognosis, and one series showed a 100% mortality rate in alcoholics with *Klebsiella pneumoniae* bacteremia despite adequate treatment with an aminoglycoside and a second- or third-generation cephalosporin.

CASE 11

History: A 52-year-old white man was hospitalized for hematemesis, diabetic ketoacidosis, and decreased mental status. A nasointestinal tube was placed to facilitate feeding. He subsequently developed fever, substernal chest pain, and respiratory distress.

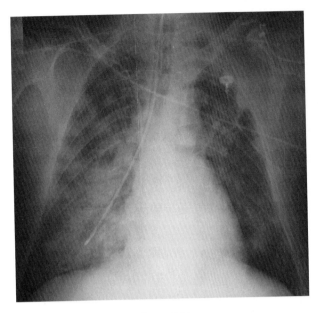

Figure 11A

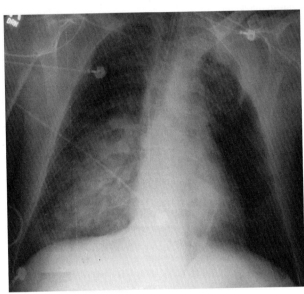

Figure 11B

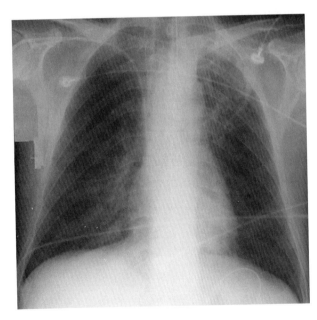

Figure 11C

Findings: Three chest radiographs taken 3 days apart are shown here. The first film shows a feeding tube placed in the right lower lobe bronchus (*A*). A fluffy focal airspace opacity surrounds the tube. The second film shows interval removal of the tube and decrease in the size of the infiltrate (*B*). A third radiograph taken several days later showed clearing of the airspace opacity in the right lower lobe following treatment (*C*).

Differential Diagnosis: A focal consolidation like this usually represents an infectious or aspiration pneumonia. However, the presence of a feeding tube in a bronchus is pathognomonic for aspiration.

Diagnosis: Aspiration pneumonia.

Discussion: Aspiration usually falls into one of three categories: aspiration of oropharyngeal secretions, aspiration of foreign bodies, or aspiration of gastric contents. Aspiration of foreign bodies is mainly seen in children. Aspiration of oropharyngeal secretions occurs in 45% of normal individuals and 70% of obtunded patients. Most do not develop pneumonia, suggesting that a defect in the normal protective mechanisms also must be present. Massive aspiration of gastric contents is termed *Mendelson's syndrome*. Risk factors include pregnancy, altered consciousness, and nasogastric intubation. Mendelson's syndrome is suggested by the abrupt onset of cough, wheezing, cyanosis, dyspnea, and tachypnea in a susceptible patient.

In Mendelson's syndrome, the aspirated gastric contents cause a chemical tracheobronchitis and pneumonia. Solid particles can obstruct the airways, leading to secondary bacterial pneumonia, abscess formation, bronchiectasis, or empyema. Pulmonary embolism and ARDS also may complicate the course. The severity of the pulmonary changes is dependent on the volume and pH of the fluid aspirated. A pH of less than 2.4 is associated with severe tracheobronchitis, necrosis of the alveolar lining, and alveolar edema and hemorrhage.

The classic radiographic appearance is diffuse perihilar alveolar consolidation. Bilateral involvement is seen in more than half of cases, although this depends on the position of the patient at the time of aspiration. Infiltrates may appear as confluent densities with air bronchograms, as 5- to 6-mm poorly defined acinar nodules, as small irregular shadows, or as a mixture of patterns. Atelectasis and pleural abnormalities are seen infrequently. Worsening of the chest radiograph over the first 36 hours is usual, but persistent worsening after 3 days or after a period of improvement suggests a complication, including bacterial pneumonia, pulmonary embolism, or acute ARDS.

CASE 12

History: The patient was an 86-year-old white woman being evaluated for a right parotid mass, with a history of occasional gurgling noises in her throat when she ate.

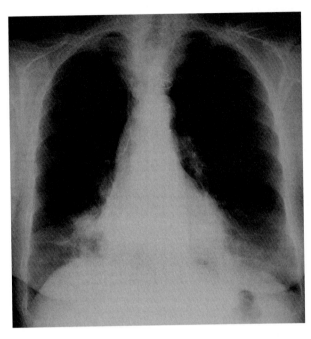

Figure 12A

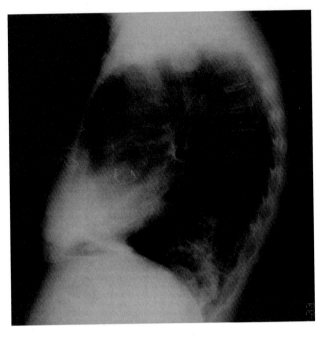

Figure 12B

Findings: PA and lateral views of the chest demonstrated bibasilar airspace disease representing aspiration pneumonia, more pronounced on the right side than on the left. Prior studies showed that these infiltrates were chronic and unchanged. In addition, increased soft tissue density was present in a paratracheal location from the Zenker's diverticulum.

Differential Diagnosis: If no previous study results had been available, pneumonia and neoplastic processes would have been included in the differential diagnosis.

Diagnosis: Aspiration pneumonia, Zenker's diverticulum.

Discussion: Zenker's diverticulum is an epithelial-lined mucosal pouch occurring at the junction of the pharynx and esophagus. It is classified as a pulsion diverticulum because it is thought to be caused by increased intraluminal pressure, often from a dysfunctional cricopharyngeus muscle. The increased intraluminal pressure causes the mucosa and submucosa to herniate through a weak point in the muscle layer, causing a false diverticulum in the area proximal to the cricopharyngeus. The prevalence of Zenker's diverticulum has been estimated at anywhere from 0.01% to 0.11% of the population, but it is more common in women and in the elderly. It is thought by some clinicians that its prevalence may be as high as 50% among individuals in their seventh and eighth decades of life.

The symptoms of Zenker's diverticulum include cervical dysphagia, effortless regurgitation of undigested food or pills, gurgling in the neck when swallowing, and, in about 30%, recurrent aspiration. Aspiration of the contents of Zenker's diverticulum leads to particle-related complications if undigested food is present. In contrast to gastric aspirate, esophageal aspirate is usually alkaline and does not cause a chemical pneumonitis. However, esophageal aspirate does contain oropharyngeal pathogens, resulting in bacterial pneumonia.

The diagnosis of Zenker's diverticulum is made by barium esophagography. It presents as a posterior midline outpouching at the pharyngoesophageal junction. The treatment of choice is excision of the diverticulum with cervical esophagomyotomy, which decreases intraluminal pressure and usually prevents relapse.

CASE 13

History: A 25-year-old white woman with AIDS complained of a 3-month history of fatigue and nonproductive cough. She had also had anorexia and temperatures of up to 103°F. Her social history was significant for a 1-year stay in a homeless shelter.

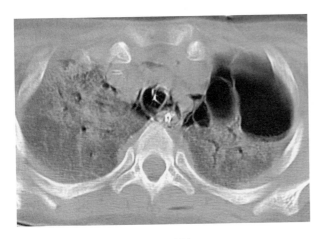

Figure 13A

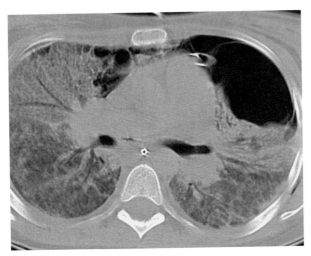

Figure 13B

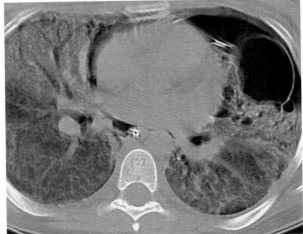

Figure 13C

Findings: CT of the chest showed diffuse bilateral airspace opacities with diffuse ground-glass changes and multiple large cystic air-filled spaces bilaterally. These were consistent with pneumatoceles. There was a large anterior pneumothorax on the left side and a small one on the right. Air was also present in the mediastinum.

Diagnosis: PCP.

Discussion: PCP is seen in patients with a CD4 count of less than $200/mm^3$ who are not on prophylaxis. In fact, before the use of prophylaxis became widespread, PCP affected 50% of all persons with AIDS at some time in the course of their disease. Prophylaxis has decreased its incidence, and effective treatment has decreased the associated mortality rate to 5% to 10%. Patients experience a prodrome of fever, malaise, and weight loss that may last several weeks. They then develop a cough productive of scant frothy white sputum, increased respiratory rate, and dyspnea on exertion.

Chest radiography shows fine bilateral perihilar reticular infiltrates or ground-glass shadowing, both of which progress to alveolar consolidation with air bronchograms in 3 to 4 days. If the infection continues, irregular coarse reticular infiltrates become visible. A small minority of patients present with a normal chest radiograph.

Pneumocystis carinii pneumonia appears as scattered airspace consolidation on high-resolution CT, varying from ground-glass to solid opacity. There is often a sharp demarcation between diseased and normal lung tissue. Interlobular septa may be thickened. Pneumatoceles are also common in the acute or post-infectious period. These thin-walled, air-containing cysts develop in about a third of acute infections. They are most commonly seen in the upper lobe, although they can develop anywhere. Pneumatoceles typically resolve spontaneously. They may be complicated by spontaneous pneumothorax.

CASE 14

History: A 55-year-old white man with a history of chronic lymphocytic leukemia and a previous history of squamous cell carcinoma of the parotid gland presented with fever, shortness of breath, and cough. He had recently been diagnosed with bacterial conjunctivitis and herpes zoster of the right face. He was found to be severely hypoxic on pulse oximetry.

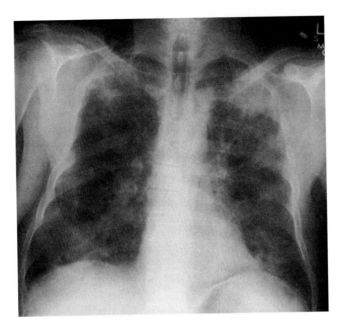

Figure 14A

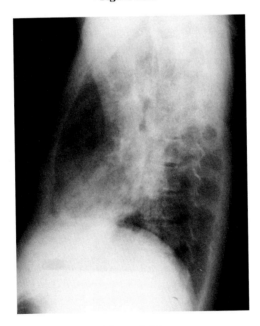

Figure 14B

Findings: PA and lateral chest radiographs were obtained and demonstrated diffuse and patchy alveolar opacities with a predominance of focal consolidation of the left upper lobe. Lateral radiography also demonstrated extensive mediastinal adenopathy with filling in of the AP window.

Differential Diagnosis: This pattern correlates with an acute pneumonia of bacterial, viral, or fungal etiology. Disseminated varicella is a consideration given the patient's immunosuppression (due to lymphoma) and history of zoster. TB can have a similar appearance in immunocompromised patients. Bronchoscopy revealed *Pneumocystis carinii* on silver stain.

Diagnosis: PCP.

Discussion: PCP is common in patients who are immunosuppressed owing to organ transplantation, hematologic malignancy, HIV infection, or an inflammatory condition requiring even low-dose steroids. Although the number of AIDS-related cases of PCP is decreasing due to improved AIDS therapy and better defined prophylaxis protocols, the incidence of non–AIDS-related cases is increasing. Non–AIDS-related PCP is associated with a higher overall mortality rate and a higher rate of hospitalization, intubation, and intensive care unit admission.

Patients with leukemia may be immunosuppressed due to the malignancy itself or due to the cytotoxic drugs used in treatment. Fludarabine, for example, is used in recurrent CLL. It causes a profound T-cell lymphopenia, which predisposes patients to *Listeria monocytogenes* meningitis and PCP. There is evidence that PCP prophylaxis may have a role in the treatment of some patients with hematologic malignancies.

CASE 15

History: A 36-year-old black man presented with fever, progressive shortness of breath, and dyspnea on exertion that had developed over the course of 3 weeks. The patient's arterial blood gases showed a P_aO_2 of 80 mmHg with an A-a gradient of 80 mmHg. Bilateral venograms showed no deep venous thromboses, and V/Q scan was negative for pulmonary embolism.

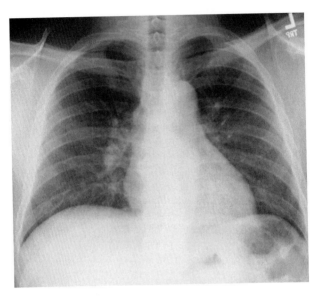

Figure 15A

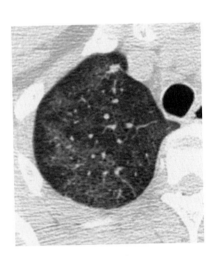

Figure 15B

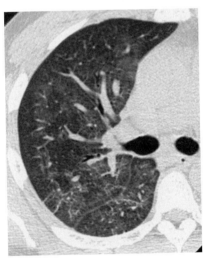

Figure 15C

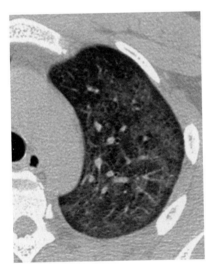

Figure 15D

Findings: Chest radiography showed only subtle cropping of the pulmonary vasculature, especially at the bases. CT of the chest showed patchy ground-glass changes throughout the lung parenchyma. There was focal consolidation within the right lower lobe and bibasilar atelectasis.

Diagnosis: PCP.

Discussion: This is another example of PCP occurring in a patient with AIDS and a CD4 count below 200 cells/mm^3. The diagnosis of PCP was confirmed through bronchoscopy. A subsequent HIV test was positive, and the CD4 count was 100 cells/mm^3. Early in the course of the AIDS epidemic, PCP was often the first presentation of HIV disease. Although this scenario is less common now due to improved awareness and testing, this case demonstrates that PCP continues to be a not uncommon presenting condition for HIV. Patients who are not known to be immunosuppressed and have clinical and radiographic evidence of PCP should be tested for HIV. Because HIV-infected patients are so susceptible to PCP, they should be placed on prophylaxis with trimethoprim/sulfamethoxazole or pentamidine if their CD4 counts fall below 200 cells/mm^3. The use of prophylaxis has reduced the 1-year incidence of PCP in this group by half.

Patients who develop PCP despite prophylaxis with aerosolized pentamidine often have atypical radiographic presentations. The pattern of diffuse infiltrates is less common, and there is an increased incidence of cysts, pneumothorax, and focal infiltrates, especially in the apical region. It was originally speculated that aerosolized pentamidine does not reach high concentrations in the apices of the lungs, making these areas susceptible, but recent research has indicated that this is not the case. However, no alternative explanation has gained support.

A significant number of patients with PCP present with a normal chest radiograph. A gallium citrate scan may be useful in these circumstances. There will be homogenous uptake throughout the lung, with a greater intensity than the liver. This is a 95% sensitive test, but it is not specific for PCP, and a positive result should be confirmed with a diagnostic procedure such as bronchoscopy.

CASE 16

History: A 37-year-old white man with a 40-pack per year history of tobacco use had a sudden onset of shortness of breath and pleuritic chest pain with subsequent development of a cough productive of white phlegm, fever, chills, night sweats, and multiple episodes of emesis secondary to the intractable cough.

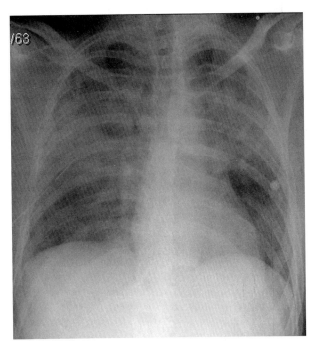

Figure 16A

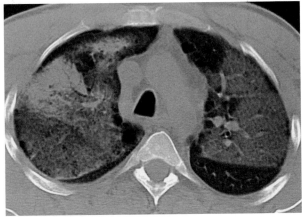

Figure 16B

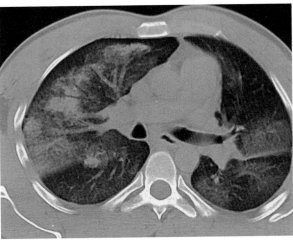

Figure 16C

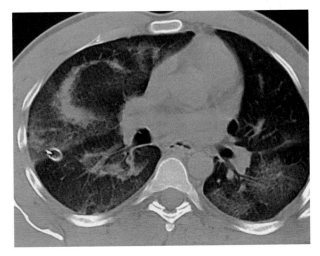

Figure 16D

Findings: Frontal chest radiography showed diffuse bilateral airspace opacities that were confluent in nature and worse in the upper lobes. CT of the chest was subsequently obtained and revealed dense upper lobe opacities with air bronchograms and diffuse ground-glass opacities throughout the lungs, but worse in the upper lobes.

Diagnosis: *Candida albicans* pneumonia.

Discussion: Bronchoscopy was performed in this patient, which revealed fungal organisms consistent with *Candida* infection. Cultures subsequently grew *Candida albicans.* All other cultures and stains were negative.

Candida pneumonia is somewhat unusual in an immunocompetent host; thus, with this presentation a further immunologic workup is needed, including HIV status. This patient was found to have no other immunologic deficiency at the time of presentation and treatment. Response to therapy is often dependent on the underlying immune status.

Candida pneumonia can present as airspace pneumonia, either as a lobar pneumonia or with multilobar involvement, or as an interstitial pneumonia. The ground-glass opacity seen is representative of acinar filling from debris or hemorrhage. Occasionally, there is an associated pleural effusion or hilar lymphadenopathy. CT findings include consolidations with air bronchograms, focal consolidation with ground-glass halo (denoting hemorrhage), and possibly hilar adenopathy and effusions.

CASE 17

History: A 69-year-old white man presented to the clinic complaining of occasional left-sided pleuritic chest pain and progressive shortness of breath for over a year. There was no radiation, diaphoresis, nausea, or vomiting. He also complained of a cough productive of yellow sputum. The patient had a history of left-sided small cell cancer several years earlier diagnosed on open lung biopsy and treated with chemotherapy and radiation therapy. All lymph nodes sampled were negative. Two weeks prior to presentation, the patient underwent another open lung biopsy, which showed extensive pulmonary fibrosis but no tumor.

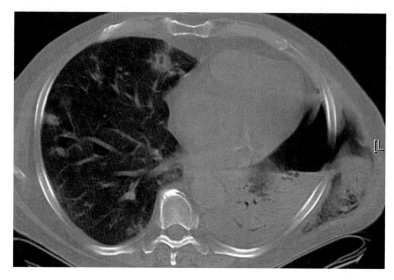

Figure 17A

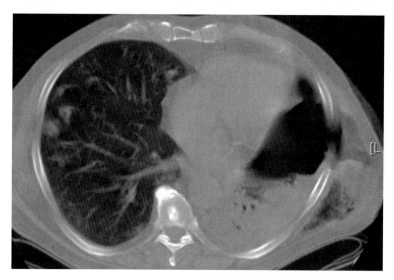

Figure 17B

Findings: Selected images from a CT scan of the chest showed a hydropneumothorax on the left side, with a fistula from the chest cavity to the subcutaneous soft tissues of the chest wall. There was extensive consolidation of the left lower lobe. Multiple 1- to 2-cm nodular densities were seen throughout the right and left lungs. There was also a significant degree of subcutaneous emphysema, which was most striking on the scout film. There was no evidence of interstitial thickening consistent with pulmonary fibrosis.

Differential Diagnosis: Nodular consolidations may represent invasive aspergillosis versus multiple pulmonary emboli. The presence of a pleural fluid collection communicating with the subcutaneous tissues can represent a variety of infectious processes, including TB, actinomycosis, and a number of pyogenic and fungal pathogens. A neoplastic process may have a similar appearance, and bronchogenic cancer, mesothelioma, and lymphoma should be considered if there is a clinical suspicion.

Diagnosis: Aspergillosis and empyema necessitans.

Discussion: Empyema necessitans is an encapsulated empyema that ruptures and drains into the surrounding soft tissues. Focal pneumonic processes predispose patients to developing empyema necessitans. In the preantibiotic era, it was most often a complication of *Mycobacterium tuberculosis* or pneumococcus pneumonia. Today most cases are due to inadequate treatment of an empyema following a necrotizing pneumonia or lung abscess. Thus, although TB is still a major pathogen, anaerobes such as *Actinomyces* are more common agents. Pyogenic organisms and fungi also have been reported as causative organisms. Invasive aspergillosis is a rare cause. Multiple factors contribute to the rupture of an empyema and subsequent dissection through the soft tissues. In many patients with empyema, there is a constant positive pressure in the pleural fluid throughout all phases of respiration. When this is combined with a weakness in the body cavity wall caused by inflammation and necrosis, rupture occurs. The most common site of a communicating fistula is in the intercostal space of the anterior chest wall, between the mid-clavicular and mid-axillary lines. However, drainage into the esophagus, bronchi, breast, mediastinum, and retroperitoneum also has been described.

CASE 18

History: A 54-year-old white man known to have large B-cell non-Hodgkin's lymphoma had undergone chemotherapy and allogenic peripheral blood stem cell transplantation from his brother. He was admitted for declining respiratory status and had gradual onset of increasing shortness of breath, new onset of atrial fibrillation, and progressive hypoxia. His respiratory status continued to decline, and he required endotracheal intubation; he eventually experienced respiratory arrest despite aggressive therapy.

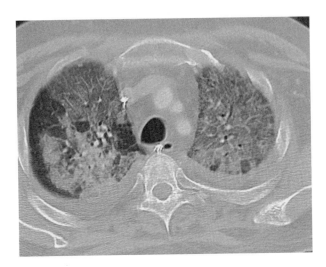

Figure 18A

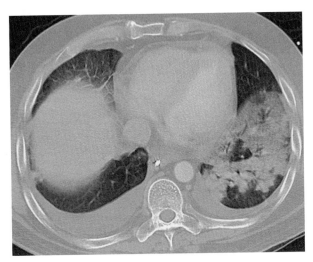

Figure 18B

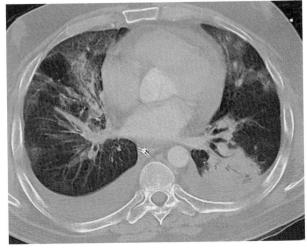

Figure 18C

Findings: CT of the chest was obtained prior to his intubation and showed diffuse ground-glass opacities throughout both lung fields with ill-defined margins and shaggy and irregular borders. More confluent areas of dense consolidation were evident with air bronchograms as well as multiple small nodular opacities and bilateral pleural effusions.

Diagnosis: Invasive aspergillosis.

Discussion: The diagnosis of invasive aspergillosis was confirmed at autopsy, unfortunately. The patient had undergone bronchoscopy that did not yield fungal elements, but he had been empirically treated since admission with aggressive antifungal therapy. The patient's underlying immunocompromised state, the degree of pulmonary parenchymal involvement, and the invasive nature of the *Aspergillus* led to his death, despite these measures. Fungal pneumonia in this patient population often has such an unfortunate outcome. In general, four distinct manifestations of aspergillus infections may be considered:

1. Mycetoma: formation of a fungus ball occurs within a preexisting cavity, most commonly the result of TB, sarcoidosis, and bullous emphysema. This situation is usually undetected unless the patient presents with hemoptysis. An opacity is seen within the dependent portion of a cavity, which shifts as the patient changes position. An "air-crescent" sign may be noted.
2. Invasive aspergillosis: occurs in the immunosuppressed host as in this patient. It has the appearance of nodular opacities, with the formation of an air-crescent sign. Diffuse, rapidly progressive consolidation also may be seen. There may be a halo of ground-glass attenuation surrounding these nodules or infiltrates, secondary to focal lung infarction/necrosis.
3. Semi-invasive aspergillosis: occurs in alcoholics, elderly debilitated patients, or patients with malignancy or radiation-damaged lungs. Formation of a mycetoma within an area of cavitation after focal parenchymal infection and necrosis is caused by the *Aspergillus* organism itself. Focal consolidation is seen initially, followed by cavitation and mycetoma formation.
4. Allergic bronchopulmonary aspergillosis: occurs in chronic asthmatics in association with bronchial mucus plugging and dilatation. On chest radiography, tubular shadows caused by dilated, mucus-filled bronchi are seen. Occasionally, a "cluster of grapes" appearance may be seen in patients with severe cystic bronchial dilatation.

CASE 19

History: A 55-year-old black man complained of right pleuritic chest pain for 5 days. He denied having fevers, chills, night sweats, or weight loss. His chronic productive cough had not changed.

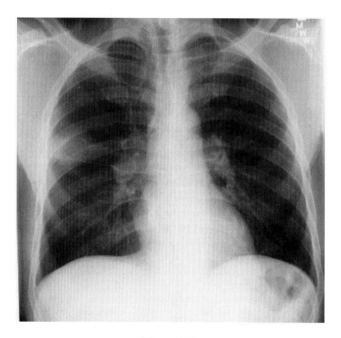

Figure 19A

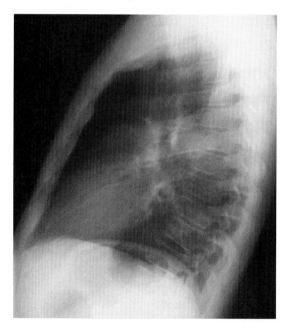

Figure 19B

Findings: PA and lateral chest radiographs were obtained. There was a 3×5 cm masslike density in the posterior right upper lobe abutting the major fissure, with consolidation also present in the superior segment of the right lower lobe.

Differential Diagnosis: Considering the sudden onset of chest pain and absence of constitutional symptoms, lung abscess is most likely. Bronchogenic cancer also should be considered. Pulmonary infarction would also be a diagnostic consideration.

Diagnosis: *Actinomyces* and *Candida* lung abscess.

Discussion: A percutaneous biopsy of the right upper lobe lesion revealed *Candida* pseudohyphae and numerous cocci and bacilli, including filamentous, anaerobic gram-positive bacilli consistent with *Actinomyces israleii.* Actinomycosis is often seen in alcoholics with poor dental hygiene. It is part of the normal flora of the mouth and oropharynx, but in susceptible tissues it causes a chronic inflammatory reaction characterized by abscesses with tiny sulfur granules in thick pus. Proteolytic enzymes produced by the bacteria allow it to cross fascial planes with ease. This accounts for its tendency to spread to the mediastinum, pleura, and chest wall. On chest radiography and CT, it appears as an area of persistent consolidation or mass, and may cavitate. Pleural involvement is usually in the form of a small pleural effusion, pleural thickening, or empyema. There is a high incidence of intrathoracic lymphadenopathy.

CASE 20

History: A 59-year-old black woman was a kidney transplant recipient with a right upper lobe pneumonia refractory to antibiotic treatment. She complained of right neck pain and a tender neck mass overlying the right lobe of the thyroid.

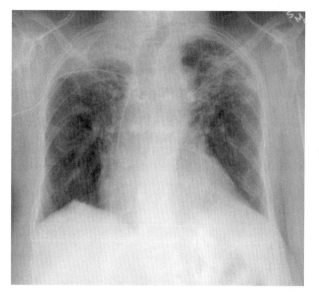

Figure 20A

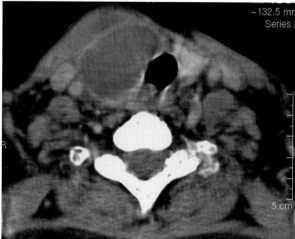

Figure 20B

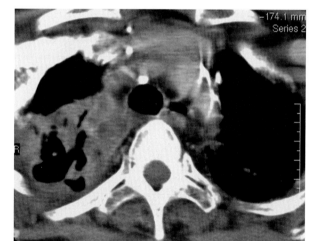

Figure 20C

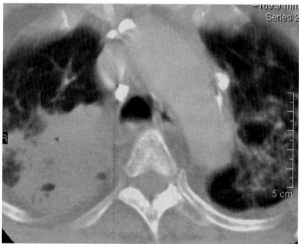

Figure 20D

Findings: PA radiograph and CT of the chest showed dense right upper lobe consolidation, with air bronchograms and central cavitation. There were small bilateral pleural effusions, and bilateral nonenlarged calcified hilar nodes. A 2.5-cm low-attenuation mass in the right anterior neck had a necrotic appearance.

Differential Diagnosis: Sputum culture was positive for *Nocardia*. Fine-needle aspiration of the neck mass revealed a purulent exudate, which proved to be *Nocardia* on Gram stain.

Diagnosis: Pulmonary nocardiosis with contiguous thyroid abscess.

Discussion: Pulmonary nocardiosis occurs when bacteria of the genus *Nocardia* (80%–90% of infections can be traced to *Nocardia asteroides*) are inhaled by a susceptible host. *Nocardia* species are common saprophytic organisms in soil and dust. They are filamentous gram-positive bacteria that stain weakly acid-fast and grow slowly on ordinary laboratory media. Nocardiosis most often presents in older adults, with a male:female ratio of 2.4:1. The incidence of reported cases has risen; this may be due to increased use of immunosuppression, although greater awareness and better diagnostic tests have contributed to the increase in the diagnosis.

One half to two thirds of patients who develop pulmonary nocardiosis have some chronic disease (PAP and COPD in particular) or are immunosuppressed. Immunosuppressed patients tend to have a worse prognosis: the mortality rate from pulmonary nocardiosis is doubled in immunosuppressed patients when compared with all others. Although there is evidence that cell-mediated immunity is an important host defense against nocardiosis, there has not been an increased incidence in nocardiosis associated with HIV. However, HIV-infected patients are prone to atypical radiographic presentations.

Clinically, pulmonary nocardiosis presents with subacute, chronic, or relapsing cough, dyspnea, and fever. In 28% to 45% of patients, the organism disseminates through the blood stream and forms distant abscesses. The central nervous system is a common site. If the patient presents with focal neurologic deficits, brain abscess should be suspected. The patient in this case had contiguous disease to her thyroid, and multiple brain abscesses were found on MRI.

On plain chest films, nocardiosis presents as a solitary or multifocal area of consolidation with patchy, lobar, or segmental distribution. Another common presentation is as a solitary nodular lesion. Cavitation is seen in almost 50% of cases, and results in thick-walled abscesses. One third of HIV-infected patients with pulmonary nocardiosis present with bilateral interstitial infiltrate. On CT, nocardiosis appears as focal nodules or focal areas of consolidation with central low attenuation.

CASE 21

History: A 45-year-old white woman had undergone bone marrow transplantation 41 days earlier for acute myelogenous leukemia. She presented to the clinic complaining of persistent high fevers. Chest x-ray showed diffuse bilateral airspace infiltrates. She was found to have CMV antigenemia and *Enterococcus cloacae* bacteremia. There was no response to treatment with antibiotics.

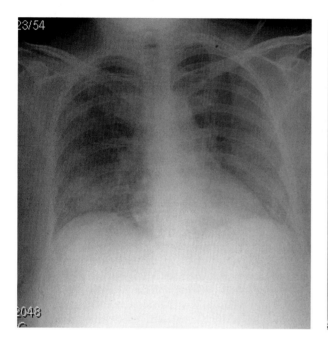

Figure 21A

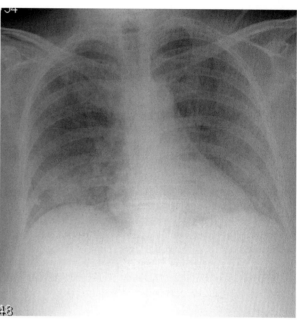

Figure 21B

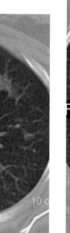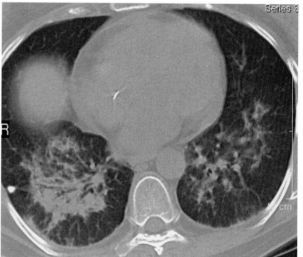

Figure 21C

Figure 21D

Findings: Two frontal views of the chest obtained several days apart showed worsening patchy bilateral airspace disease. CT showed diffuse bilateral central airspace disease, with some acinar filling giving a tree-and-bud appearance (*C*).

Differential Diagnosis: This pattern could represent an atypical bacterial, viral, or fungal pneumonia. British anti-Lewisite was positive for CMV inclusion bodies.

Diagnosis: CMV pneumonia.

Discussion: Human CMV infection is a common complication of bone marrow transplantation, with clinical or subclinical infections occurring in up to 70% of recipients. It presents as retinitis, esophagitis, hepatitis, nephritis, or enterocolitis, usually in the first 30 to 100 days following transplantation. Pneumonia is another common presentation, seen in 10% to 40% of allogenic transplant recipients, and is responsible for most of the morbidity and mortality associated with this pathogen. Diagnosis of CMV pneumonia requires bronchoalveolar lavage or lung biopsy demonstrating CMV cellular inclusion bodies. Early diagnosis and treatment with ganciclovir can cut the mortality rate by half.

Cytomegalovirus often presents on chest radiographs as reticular or reticulonodular infiltrates with a predilection for the lung bases. It also can present as confluent airspace disease, or even with a normal x-ray. A CT pattern of focal basilar consolidation or multiple small nodules is suggestive of CMV pneumonia, but areas of ground-glass consolidation and reticular infiltrates may be seen.

CASE 22

History: A 26-year-old woman had a 3-week history of a nonproductive cough, as well as shortness of breath and left-sided pleuritic chest pain. She admitted to fevers, chills, and night sweats, and had lost 5 pounds over the 3 months prior to admission. She had no hemoptysis and recalled no TB contacts. She was a native of India and came to the United States 3 years earlier. She worked in a microbiology laboratory at a medical center and stated that she frequently used oral suction to pipette specimens. She had no improvement when treated with amoxicillin clavulanate.

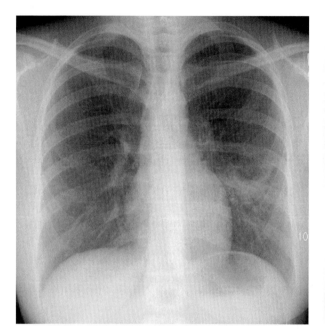

Figure 22A

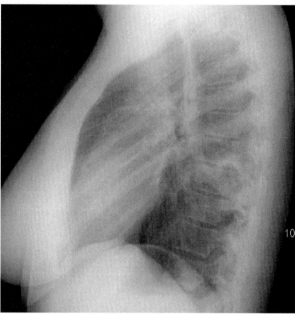

Figure 22B

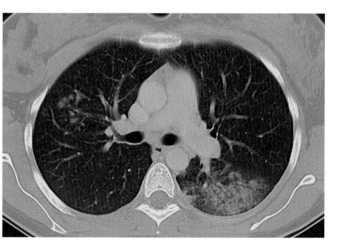

Figure 22C

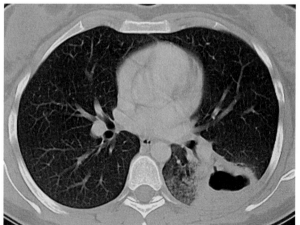

Figure 22D

Findings: PA and lateral chest radiographs showed left lower lobe consolidation. CT of the chest showed a 5-cm area of cavitation in the superior segment of the left lower lobe. There was also patchy acinar filling evident in the right lung.

Differential Diagnosis: For cavitary pneumonia that does not respond to standard antibiotics, the differential diagnosis includes TB, atypical mycobacteria, nocardiosis, and fungal pneumonia, including coccidioidomycosis. Sputum cultures grew out *Mycobacterium tuberculosis*.

Diagnosis: TB pneumonia.

Discussion: TB is epidemiologically an urban disease, and is common in prisons as well as in indigent and homeless populations. Immigrants from parts of the world where TB is endemic, such as this patient, are an important source of new cases in the United States. HIV-positive patients are at high risk for reactivation of TB, especially when their CD4 counts fall below 200 cells/mm^3. Due to senile decrease in function of the immune system, people over 65 years of age are also at high risk. Primary and reactivation TB can have a variety of radiographic appearances, including airspace infiltrates.

Although primary TB cases were typically seen in children in the past, the AIDS epidemic has resulted in an increase in the number of cases of primary TB in adults. The most common radiographic feature is unilateral hilar adenopathy, which may or may not be accompanied by a focal infiltrate. TB lymphadenopathy has a characteristic CT appearance of a central area of low attenuation surrounded by a rim of enhancement. Although lymphadenopathy can appear without infiltrate half of the time, infiltrates are almost never seen without lymphadenopathy. When an infiltrate is present, it can take on a variety of appearances, including interstitial shadowing and lobar consolidation. A normal chest x-ray is seen in 10% of cases, and is more common in patients with lower CD4 counts. Lower CD4 counts are also associated with an increased incidence of intrathoracic adenopathy, focal middle and lower lobe infiltrates, and reticulonodular or interstitial infiltrates.

Reactivation TB has a classic predilection for the posterior aspects of the upper lobes and the superior segments of the lower lobes. The airspace pattern seen in reactivation begins with a patchy consolidation with indistinct margins that may spread to involve the entire lobe. Cavitation and pleural effusion are common accompanying features. The disease spreads throughout the lungs via the airway, creating a bronchoalveolar pattern of small, patchy infiltrates bilaterally.

CASE 23

History: This patient was a 54-year-old black woman with a history of myocardial infarction 8 months prior to examination and idiopathic pulmonary fibrosis diagnosed 2 years prior to examination. She presented to the clinic with one week of worsening cough, shortness of breath, and dyspnea on exertion.

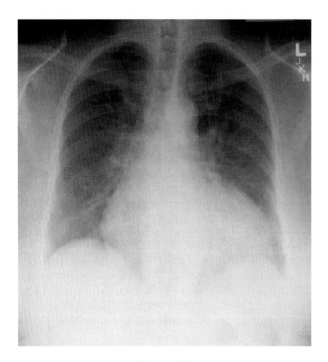

Figure 23A

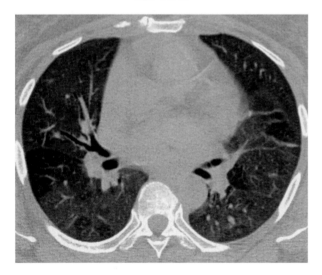

Figure 23B

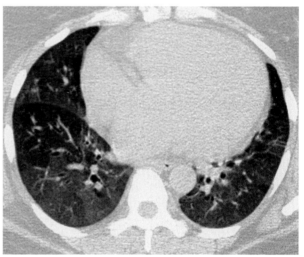

Figure 23C

Findings: On PA radiography and CT of the chest, the cardiac silhouette demonstrated moderate to severe enlargement. The lung parenchyma had a ground-glass appearance without parenchymal nodules or thickening of the interstitium. The pulmonary veins were mildly enlarged, and there was no bronchiectasis.

Diagnosis: Cardiogenic pulmonary edema.

Discussion: A variety of findings are seen on high resolution CT in cardiogenic pulmonary edema. One common finding is ground-glass opacities, which are regions of increased lung attenuation that do not obscure underlying vessels. These can be diffuse or patchy and geographic. They are caused by minimal thickening of the pulmonary interstitium or intraalveolar fluid layering against the alveolar wall. Interlobular septal thickening is another common sign. The edema fluid in the interstitium causes the appearance of linear or reticular opacities 1 to 5 mm thick. They are generally smooth and uniform, although prominent septal veins can cause focal nodularities. Pulmonary edema can cause peribronchiovascular thickening, which has a predominantly central distribution. The diameter of the pulmonary arteries and veins is increased, especially in the perihilar regions. The bronchial vessels can be used as comparisons. Finally, pleural effusions are common in severe pulmonary edema, and subpleural fluid accumulations can give the interlobar fissures a thickened appearance.

It is difficult to differentiate cardiogenic from noncardiogenic pulmonary edema based solely on radiographic findings. However, there are certain plain film features that are more suggestive of one or the other. Infiltrates that are predominantly central in distribution and appear coincidentally with the onset of symptoms suggest a cardiogenic cause, whereas a delay in the appearance of shadows and a uniform zonal distribution are more typical of ARDS. Peribronchial cuffing, septal lines, and pleural effusions are common in cardiogenic pulmonary edema, but are rarely visible in noncardiogenic forms. On the other hand, air bronchograms are seen three times as often in ARDS. Finally, some clinicians suggest that in ventilated supine patients, a cardiothoracic ratio of greater than 0.52 and a vascular pedicle wider than 63 mm suggest a hydrostatic cardiogenic edema.

CASE 24

History: A 47-year-old white man with nonischemic dilated cardiomyopathy due to hypertension was admitted for worsening symptoms of congestive heart failure, chest congestion, and cough productive of brown sputum.

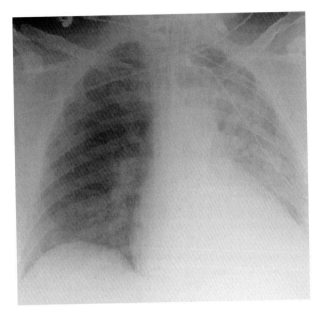

Figure 24A

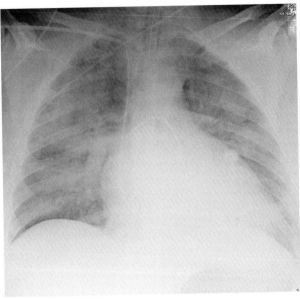

Figure 24B

Findings: Two serial chest radiographs were obtained over a 1 day interval and showed an enlarged cardiac silhouette with rapidly worsening bilateral perihilar infiltrates.

Diagnosis: Cardiogenic pulmonary edema.

Discussion: Cardiogenic pulmonary edema is mainly caused by heart disease, overhydration, or fluid retention due to renal failure. Patients present with dyspnea, orthopnea, and occasionally with expectoration of pink foam. Pathologically, the increase in intravascular volume leads to elevation of pulmonary venous and arterial pressures. Fluid first collects in the interstitium, with subsequent edema of the alveolar spaces. The radiographic findings in pulmonary edema reflect these pathologic processes and can be divided into interstitial and alveolar signs. Interstitial pulmonary edema may be seen without an alveolar component, but alveolar edema always has an interstitial component, whether radiographic signs are seen or not.

Radiographic changes correlate well with increases in PAWP. Mild increases in PAWP, below 18 mm Hg, cause redistribution of blood flow to the upper lobes. The diameter of vessels in the upper zone will be equal to or greater than the equivalent lower zone vessels. At wedge pressures of 18 to 22 mm Hg, the outer zone vessels become prominent. Also, a perihilar haze develops. The hilar and pulmonary vessels become indistinct due to interstitial fluid accumulation. At a PAWP of 22 to 25 mm Hg, fluid leaks into the alveolar spaces, creating peri-acinar rosettes on plain films. These are caused by periacinar fluid transudation, resulting in a cluster of radiolucent areas surrounded by areas of water density, suggesting a flowerlike formation.

CASE 25

History: The patient was a 20-year-old restrained driver in a motor vehicle collision.

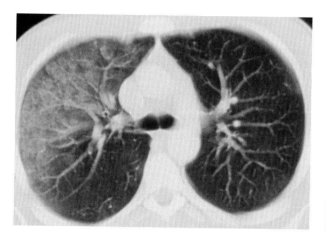

Figure 25A

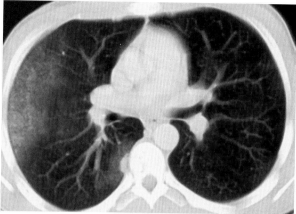

Figure 25B

Findings: CT scan of the chest revealed extensive right-sided airspace consolidation consistent with acinar filling, and ground-glass changes were noted. There was no effusion or pneumothorax.

Diagnosis: Pulmonary contusion.

Discussion: Pulmonary contusion is a common injury seen in the context of blunt thoracic trauma, and is often associated with pneumothorax, pleural effusion, and rib fractures. It manifests on chest radiography as ill-defined patchy or confluent airspace filling that appears within 6 hours of injury. Lobar and segmental patterns are generally not seen. There is usually no worsening of appearance over time, and infiltrates are marked by rapid resolution.

Chest radiographs often lag behind or do not correlate with the clinical course. Hypoxia is the best indicator of severity. If the hypoxia is particularly serious, mechanical ventilation may be indicated.

Although chest radiographs reveal most contusions, CT is even more sensitive in identifying infiltrates. A CT also may reveal pneumatoceles created by shearing of lung parenchyma and collection of air in the spaces created. If the space fills with blood, a lung hematoma results. This complication takes several weeks to resolve and may resemble cavitation on plain radiographs and CT.

CASE 26

History: A 41-year-old black man with a history of hepatitis C and alcoholism was admitted for end-stage liver disease. He underwent a TIPS procedure but continued to have liver failure and hypoalbuminemia, subsequently developing acute renal failure.

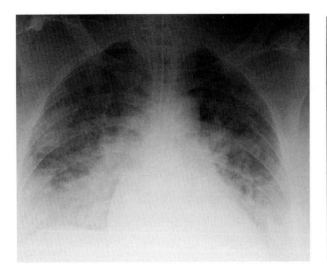

Figure 26A

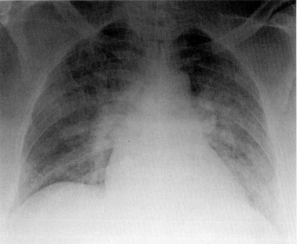

Figure 26B

Findings: Two serial chest radiographs were obtained several days apart. The first film demonstrated bilateral airspace consolidation in the lower lobes. A subsequent film showed partial clearing of the areas of consolidation, with significant airspace opacity still persisting in the left lower lobe.

Differential Diagnosis: Pulmonary edema, diffuse hemorrhage, diffuse pneumonia, and ARDS are diagnostic considerations.

Diagnosis: Pulmonary hemorrhage.

Discussion: Pulmonary hemorrhage is suggested by the presence of pulmonary consolidations in a patient with hemoptysis and anemia. Solitary airspace shadows from hemorrhage are usually due to pulmonary embolism or pulmonary contusion. They can be of any shape, including lobar. When caused by systemic disease, hemorrhage is usually multifocal. Some etiologies include Goodpasture's syndrome, ANCA-associated small vessel vasculitides, collagen vascular diseases, idiopathic pulmonary hemosiderosis, and certain drugs and chemicals. Pulmonary hemorrhage also can be seen in instances of coagulopathy, especially when the prothrombin time is greater than 20 seconds or platelet count less than 100,000 cells/mm^3. In this patient, the prothrombin time was 27 seconds and the platelet count was 20,000 cells/mm^3. It is presumed that coagulopathy was the cause of these findings.

The main radiographic finding in diffuse alveolar hemorrhage is airspace consolidation, ranging from acinar shadowing, to patchy airspace opacity, to widespread confluent consolidations with air bronchograms. The costophrenic angles and apices are usually spared. The consolidations clear in 2 to 3 days. Pleural effusions are not uncommon, but most are a secondary phenomenon related to fluid overload or infection.

CASE 27

History: A 44-year-old with Crohn's disease and a history of recurrent pneumonias presented with a 2-week history of malaise and cough, and worsening dyspnea, fevers, chills, and sweats over the preceding 2 days. The white blood cell count was 26,000 cells/μL, with 76% polymorphonuclear cells and 20% bands.

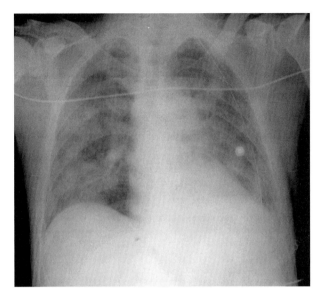

Figure 27A

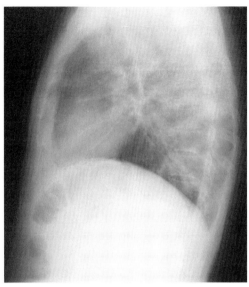

Figure 27B

Findings: PA and lateral views of the chest showed diffuse bilateral airspace disease.

Differential Diagnosis: Open lung biopsy pathology was consistent with hypersensitivity pneumonia.

Diagnosis: Hypersensitivity pneumonia.

Discussion: Hypersensitivity pneumonitis can occur as a result of drug reaction or other offending agents. Drugs that are known to cause a hypersensitivity reaction in certain individuals include nitrofurantoin, penicillin, sulfonamides, erythromycin, bleomycin, and methotrexate, among others.

   The radiographic presentation with hypersensitivity pneumonitis resembles that of eosinophilic pneumonia. Acinar filling with eosinophilic infiltrates is evident as patchy airspace opacities, often seen in the periphery of the lung. Peripheral eosinophilia may be present as well. The areas of involvement appear acutely after exposure to the offending agent and may clear rapidly only to appear in other subsegmental areas of the lung. Diffuse pulmonary edema may be present in addition, particularly with repeat exposure to an offending agent, and can occur in the hyperacute setting. The diagnosis is usually made with transbronchial tissue sampling. Response to therapy is often very dramatic, with marked improvement after treatment with corticosteroids.

CASE 28

History: A 40-year-old white man presented with fatigue, sore throat, and a temperature of 103°F. He denied having cough, nausea, or vomiting. He had been previously admitted for fatigue, hemoptysis, and advanced renal dysfunction. During that hospitalization, he was found to be positive for anti-GBM antibodies. Renal biopsy revealed glomerular crescents.

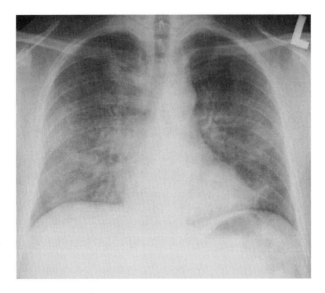

Figure 28A

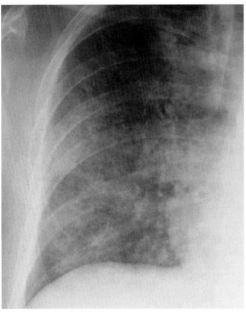

Figure 28B

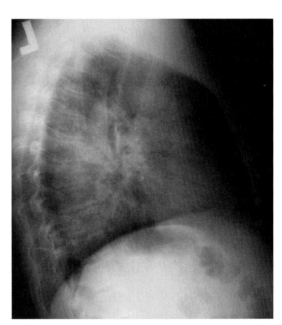

Figure 28C

Findings: There were diffuse bilateral alveolar infiltrates on the PA and lateral chest radiographs. These were better seen on the accompanying coned down view from the PA chest (*B*).

Diagnosis: Goodpasture's syndrome.

Discussion: Anti-GBM disease is divided into two categories: Goodpasture's syndrome, in which there is diffuse alveolar hemorrhage and glomerulonephritis, and Goodpasture's disease, in which there is only glomerulonephritis. The autoantibodies that are present are directed against an epitope of the type IV collagen in the basement membrane. The syndrome usually presents in young white men in their twenties or thirties. Smoking, hydrocarbon exposure, and viral infection are predisposing conditions. Patients present with hemoptysis, dyspnea, fatigue, or iron deficiency anemia. Although respiratory problems are the main presenting complaints, 80% of patients have proteinuria or hematuria at presentation.

Laboratory findings that suggest the diagnosis include a negative c-ANCA and positive anti-GBM antibodies. In that context, a renal biopsy showing subacute proliferative glomerulonephritis and linear immunoglobulin G deposition in the glomeruli is diagnostic. Lung biopsy is usually not necessary.

Treatment involves the use of steroids and immunosuppressives. Plasmapheresis may be indicated in severe cases. Renal failure requires supportive therapy, including dialysis.

The radiologic appearance of Goodpasture's syndrome is typical for diffuse alveolar hemorrhage. Consolidation may be widespread or perihilar and patchy to confluent. Infiltrates generally resolve in less than a week.

CASE 29

History: A 68-year-old white man with a history of hypothyroidism and depression had been admitted and treated for symptoms of pneumonia three times during the preceding year. The patient presented again complaining of hemoptysis and shortness of breath. While in the hospital, his shortness of breath progressed to respiratory failure requiring intubation. He was also diagnosed with chronic renal failure, and dialysis was initiated.

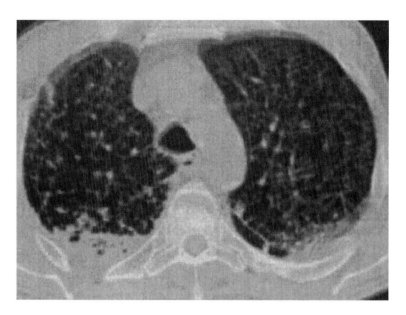

Figure 29

Findings: CT of the chest showed diffuse interstitial disease, with the right lung more extensively involved than the left. Multiple nodules were seen on the right side, the largest one being 1.5 cm in diameter. There were areas of solid consolidation in the dependent areas of the right and left lungs. The apices exhibited mild bullous disease.

Differential Diagnosis: Laboratory studies for anti-GBM antibodies were negative. Lung biopsy showed vasculitis of the capillaries and a positive p-ANCA.

Diagnosis: Wegener's granulomatosis.

Discussion: Wegener's granulomatosis is a disease characterized by necrotizing granulomatous inflammation of the upper and lower respiratory tracts, small vessel vasculitis of the arteries and veins, and focal necrotizing glomerulonephritis. It is an uncommon disease that generally affects middle-aged individuals. There is a slight male predominance. Patients usually present with nonspecific signs such as fever, malaise, weight loss, arthralgias, and chronic rhinitis. Nasal or oral mucosal ulcerations, which may cause a bloody discharge, are common. Pulmonary involvement may be asymptomatic or may cause hemoptysis, dyspnea, or chest pain. Functional renal impairment is only seen in 10% at initial presentation. Laboratory findings include anemia, leukocytosis, positive rheumatoid factor, and increased erythrocyte sedimentation rate. c-ANCA is present in 85% of patients with active disease. p-ANCA is seen in a minority of patients with Wegener's granulomatosis, but is more closely associated with polyarteritis nodosa.

Involvement of the lungs consists of inflammatory lesions, including microabscesses, suppurative granulomas, and large necrotic areas. These lesions manifest on plain films as discrete focal opacities varying from nodular masses to ill-defined areas of consolidation. Mixed patterns are also seen. Most radiographs show nodules, which are commonly 2 to 4 cm in diameter. They are usually multiple but may be single. A third of patients have focal opacities that look like consolidation. They can be single or multiple and have patchy to segmental distribution. Cavitation is seen in both types of lesions. The cavity wall will be thick initially but thins over time. Diffuse alveolar hemorrhage is seen in 8% at presentation, and appears as diffuse bilateral consolidation.

High-resolution CT of the chest in a patient with Wegener's granulomatosis shows multiple nodules 2 to 3 mm or larger in diameter. Cavitation is seen in nodules that are greater than 2 cm across. Consolidations are also seen and are pleural based. They may or may not have air bronchograms. Peribronchiovascular thickening is common. Tracheal narrowing, usually subglottic, is seen in as many as one fifth of patients. It may be symptomatic, producing dyspnea, hoarseness, and stridor.

CASE 30

History: A 70-year-old white man with a prior history of a renal transplant presented with a 3-day history of increasing shortness of breath, fevers, and chills. PA and lateral chest radiographs and CT were obtained.

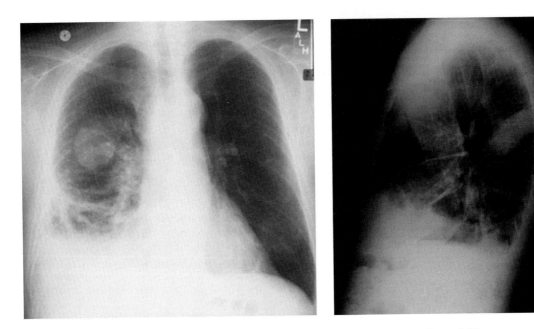

Figure 30A

Figure 30B

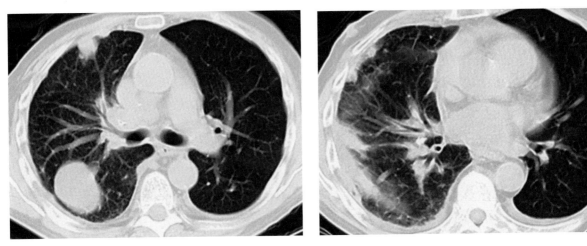

Figure 30C

Figure 30D

Findings: PA and lateral chest radiographs demonstrated a large opacity in the right lung, which the lateral film showed to be overlying the fissure. There was also a right-sided pleural effusion with associated atelectasis in the right lung and areas of patchy opacity in both lung bases. CT showed several pulmonary parenchymal masses that were subsequently submitted for biopsy for diagnostic purposes, as were the fluid and masslike density within the pleural space.

Diagnosis: PAP with pulmonary nocardiosis.

Discussion: PAP predisposes patients to a variety of infectious processes, with *Nocardia asteroides, Mycobacterium tuberculosis, Pneumocystis carinii,* and *Mycobacterium avium intracellulare* being especially common pathogens. High fever in the setting of PAP suggests superinfection, often by one of these agents.

The prognosis of PAP is variable. About one third of cases resolve spontaneously or respond to therapy quickly. One third of patients have a recurrent course with repeated attacks over the years. And one third of patients have a poor prognosis. Treatment of PAP consists of repeated lobar lavage.

The large opacity seen in the right hemithorax is representative of a pseudotumor. This is representative of fluid seen within the major fissure on the right. CT reveals multiple smaller areas of airspace opacity, which have a predominantly peripheral distribution. Fungal disease or atypical infections and septic emboli often present with this appearance of multiple peripheral ill-defined pulmonary parenchymal nodules. This patient is particularly susceptible to unusual infections secondary to immunosuppression for his renal transplant.

CASE 31

History: A 45-year-old woman had a long history of recurrent bouts of hemoptysis, cough, and worsening dyspnea on exertion.

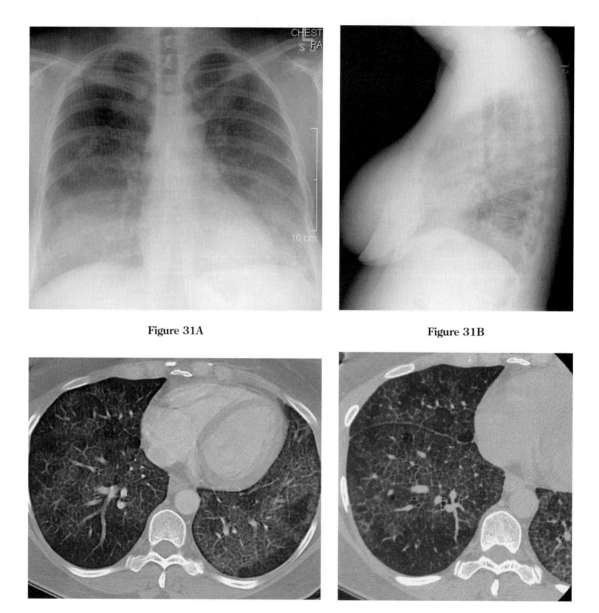

Figure 31A

Figure 31B

Figure 31C

Figure 31D

Findings: PA and lateral chest radiographs showed hazy opacification of both lungs, particularly involving the lower lobes. CT of the chest with thin section high-resolution images showed ground-glass attenuation within both lungs diffusely as well as prominent and thickened interlobular septae.

Diagnosis: Alveolar proteinosis.

Discussion: Alveolar proteinosis typically presents as insidious onset of progressive dyspnea and cough in a 30- to 50-year-old man. Patients also may complain of pleuritic chest pain, hemoptysis, hypoxemia, clubbing, or crepitation. Less common is an acute presentation with dyspnea, fever, and weight loss. Laboratory findings consistent with the diagnosis include elevation of serum apoproteins A and B and lactate dehydrogenase levels.

Alveolar proteinosis can be a primary process or can occur secondary to chemical exposure, infection, or immunocompromise. It probably represents a response of the lung to injury. The air spaces fill with a surfactant-like proteinaceous fluid that contains cellular debris. Chest radiographs show bilateral symmetric perihilar airspace opacity. The opacities are finely granular or made of coarse acinar nodules. Pathologically, the interstitium is not involved, although septal fibrosis and edema may be seen radiographically. The characteristic CT finding in alveolar proteinosis is "crazy paving." This term refers to the marked reticular pattern superimposed on areas of ground-glass opacity, caused by thickening of the interlobular and intralobular septa. This pattern is well demonstrated in this case. Superinfection by bacteria, fungi, and viruses is relatively common and is suggested by the findings of local consolidation denser than ground-glass, cavitation, or pulmonary effusion. Alveolar proteinosis clears spontaneously in one fourth to one third of patients, but most patients require treatment with saline lavage to aid recovery. (Case courtesy of Dr. Mark Brantly.)

CASE 32

History: A 36-year-old white man with diabetes mellitus presented with 6 weeks of progressive shortness of breath and nonproductive cough. He had been having fevers of up to 100°F. He had also lost 25 pounds over the previous 3 weeks. Oxygen saturation at admission was 83%.

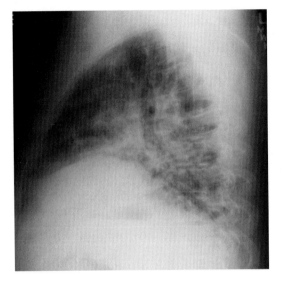

Figure 32A

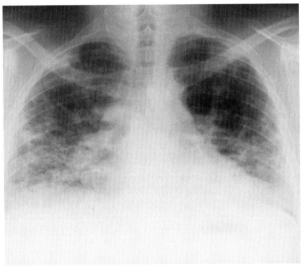

Figure 32B

Findings: PA and lateral chest radiographs showed diffuse bilateral interstitial disease that was worse at the bases. There was patchy consolidation of both lower lobes.

Differential Diagnosis: Several infectious processes can give this appearance, as can organizing pneumonia. Pulmonary edema is an unlikely etiology given this presentation.

Diagnosis: BOOP.

Discussion: In BOOP, there is patchy cellular fibrosis that fills and occludes bronchioles, alveolar ducts, and alveoli. It is classified into primary, secondary, and focal varieties. Primary organizing pneumonia is seen in middle-aged patients of either sex. Clinically, there is an influenza-like prodrome that is followed by several weeks of cough, dyspnea, malaise, fever, and weight loss. Chest radiographs show bilateral patchy airspace opacity that may be of ground-glass density. The consolidation has a peribronchial and peripheral distribution. Nodular densities are also occasionally seen. CT shows multifocal subpleural consolidations that may be of ground-glass density. Air bronchograms are common. Opacities tend to be bilateral but have an asymmetric distribution.

Some causes of secondary organizing pneumonia include infection, collagen vascular diseases, and hematologic malignancies. Secondary BOOP is in all aspects identical to the primary form, but carries a worse prognosis.

Focal organizing pneumonia is usually asymptomatic and appears as an incidental finding of a solitary nodule on chest radiographs. The prognosis is generally very good. On CT, the lesion may appear as a small irregular mass with a pleural tag or as a larger oval lesion with broad pleural contact.

CASE 33

History: A 45-year-old white man with a history of COPD and alcoholic cirrhosis presented with fever, productive cough, and shortness of breath that progressed to respiratory distress, requiring intubation. He had a 40 pack year smoking history.

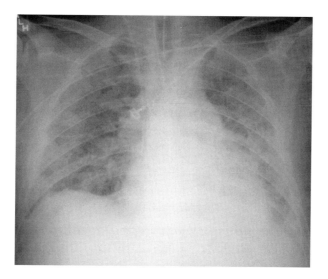

Figure 33

Findings: A frontal view of the chest showed bilateral diffuse nodular areas of consolidation that have a nonspecific appearance.

Differential Diagnosis: The differential diagnosis includes diffuse inflammation and a variety of infectious etiologies. Open lung biopsy revealed BOOP.

Diagnosis: BOOP.

Discussion: In BOOP, there is patchy cellular fibrosis that fills and occludes bronchioles, alveolar ducts, and alveoli. It is classified into primary, secondary, and focal varieties.

Primary BOOP may be difficult to differentiate from infectious pneumonia based on radiographic appearance alone. Chest radiographs show bilateral patchy alveolar infiltrates of ground-glass density in 81% of patients. The consolidation has a peribronchial and peripheral distribution. Cavitation and effusions are rarely present. Nodular densities are occasionally seen. CT shows multifocal airspace consolidations in all lung zones that may be of ground-glass density. A pattern of subpleural predominance is seen in about 60%. Air bronchograms are common. Opacities tend to be bilateral but have an asymmetric distribution. CT also shows mediastinal lymphadenopathy in one-third of patients.

CASE 34

History: This patient was a 47-year-old woman with a history of recent worsening of shortness of breath and cough.

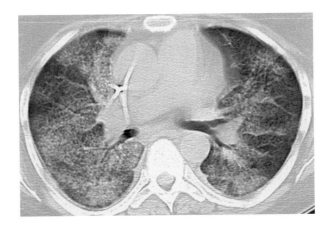

Figure 34A

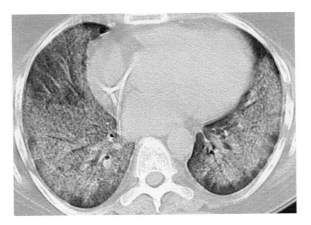

Figure 34B

Findings: Images from a CT of the chest showed diffuse mixed airspace and interstitial disease with ground-glass changes and a coarse reticular pattern of interstitial changes.

Diagnosis: BOOP.

Discussion: This is another example of BOOP demonstrating its appearance on CT. The airspace opacities are bilateral and asymmetric, and air bronchograms are present. This patient belongs in the small subset of patients who also have marked interstitial changes.

CASE 35

History: A previously healthy 32-year-old black man complained of hemoptysis ever since he was released from prison 2 weeks earlier.

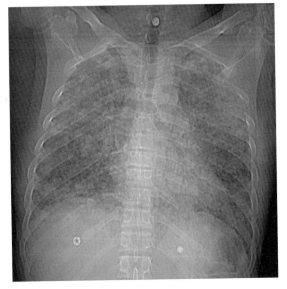

Figure 35A

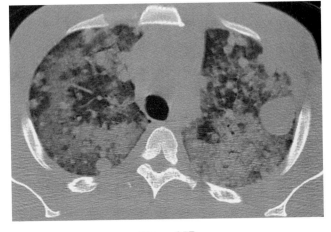

Figure 35B

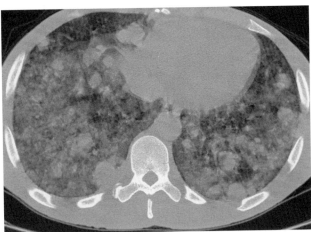

Figure 35C

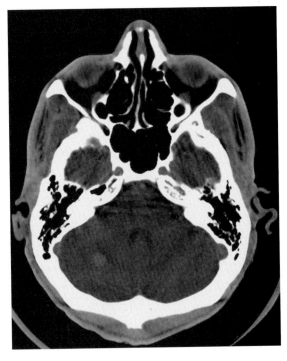

Figure 35D

Findings: A chest CT and scout topogram image demonstrated diffuse bilateral airspace disease consisting of innumerable nodules. The lung was nearly replaced with diffuse nodules, the largest measuring approximately 3 cm in diameter. There was also anterior mediastinal, prevascular, and subcarinal adenopathy. CT of the head showed a hyperdense mass in the posterior fossa on the right.

Differential Diagnosis: The pattern of nodular disease in this patient likely represents a neoplastic cause, possibly lymphoma or diffuse metastases. This radiologic pattern, in a patient with hemoptysis, should also alert the clinician to the possibility of TB or fungal infection. This patient's serum human chorionic gonadotropin (hCG) was 540,000 mIU/mL. Testicular ultrasonography showed no masses.

Diagnosis: Metastatic choriocarcinoma.

Discussion: Choriocarcinoma can appear in the lung as a metastasis or as a primary lung lesion. In metastatic disease, the primary tumor is gestational trophoblastic disease in women and testicular cancer in men. In all of these cases, elevated serum levels of β-hCG is an important marker. β-hCG levels of greater than 50,000 mIU/mL are associated with a poor prognosis.

The lung is the most common site of metastases for primary occurrences of choriocarcinoma in other parts of the body. Early in the disease, patients are asymptomatic and lung metastases present as incidental findings on chest radiographs. Later in the course of the disease, patients may develop choriocarcinoma syndrome, a distinct presentation of hemorrhage at the site of metastases, sometimes associated with thyrotoxicosis, in patients with a high volume of choriocarcinoma metastases. Radiographically, one or more pulmonary nodules with hemorrhagic infiltrate are seen in the outer portions of the lungs.

Primary choriocarcinoma of the lungs is a rare entity presenting in patients in their twenties and thirties. There is a male predominance. Other rare primary sites include the mediastinum, bladder, prostate, and pineal gland. Symptoms include scanty hemoptysis, a general decrease in health, gynectomastia, testicular atrophy, and decreased libido. On chest radiography, a nodule surrounded by diffuse shadowing is a common finding. Patients often present with hemoptysis when they have lung parenchymal metastasis, as this patient did. Brain metastases are also relatively common. Unfortunately, at the time of presentation this patient's disease was so extensive that it was poorly responsive to therapy and he died within 24 hours of admission.

CASE 36

History: A 43-year-old white woman with a history of Crohn's disease, depression, and chronic low back pain presented with a persistent right middle lobe infiltrate. The infiltrate was initially noted 6 weeks prior to presentation on a preoperative film for repair of a bulging lower back disk. She complained of worsening productive cough and subjective fevers over the preceding few weeks. Her sputum was greenish yellow. She denied having dyspnea, hemoptysis, or weight loss. She kept several birds in her house, and had a positive antibody titer for *Chlamydia psittaci*.

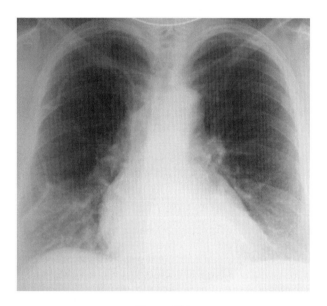

Figure 36A

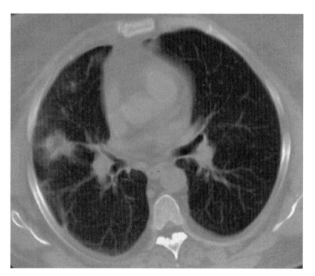

Figure 36B

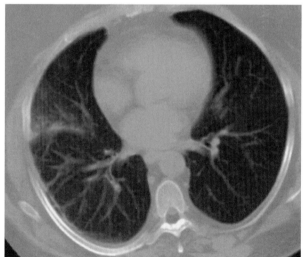

Figure 36C

Findings: An airspace pattern right middle lobe opacity was seen on chest radiography. CT showed a 2-cm mass in the right middle lobe near the minor fissure, with central low attenuation from necrosis as well as ill-defined margins and surrounding ground-glass opacity.

Differential Diagnosis: This finding is worrisome for bronchogenic carcinoma. The peripheral location makes adenocarcinoma and BAC more likely. A variety of infectious etiologies can have a similar appearance. Psittacosis is more likely to present with patchy consolidation or a patchy reticular pattern. A percutaneous CT-guided lung biopsy was performed.

Diagnosis: BAC.

Discussion: BAC is a not uncommon type of adenocarcinoma thought to arise from type II pneumocytes and bronchiolar epithelial cells. It is not associated with cigarette smoking and does not have a gender predominance. It is seen in patients 55 to 65 years of age, and has a tendency to arise out of previously damaged or scarred lung tissue. The presenting complaint may be expectoration of large amounts of mucoid sputum produced by the tumor cells. This is termed *bronchorrhea.*

Bronchioloalveolar carcinoma most commonly presents as a solitary lobulated or spiculated nodule, often in a subpleural location. Air bronchograms and bubble-like lucencies are often seen on CT, representing patent small bronchi. When it presents as a solitary nodule, it is more likely to be at stage I and is probably slow growing; the prognosis is relatively favorable.

Bronchioloalveolar carcinoma also can present as unifocal or multifocal areas of pulmonary consolidation. They may have any appearance, from ground-glass opacity to solid consolidation, with lobar to patchy, multifocal distribution. Pneumonia, aspiration, and pulmonary edema should be considered in the differential diagnosis. On CT, air bronchograms are common. As in the nodular form, a bubbly pattern of small, rounded collections of air due to patent bronchi and cystic spaces may be seen. Thickened septal lines, branching tubular densities, and mucoid impaction suggest lymphatic permeation. Pleural effusions and hilar and mediastinal lymphadenopathy are common. When BAC presents as pulmonary consolidation, local spread is more extensive, and metastasis is more common, resulting in a worse prognosis.

CASE 37

History: A 50-year-old previously healthy white man had an asymptomatic right lower lung nodule found on routine chest radiography. He had a history of tobacco use. He was scheduled for CT for further workup.

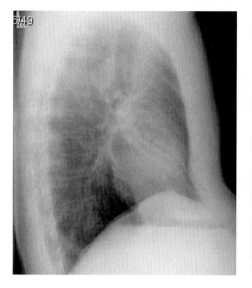

Figure 37A

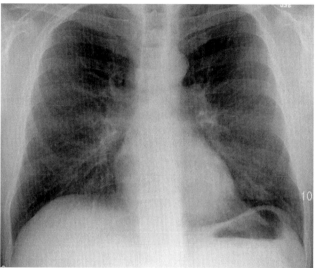

Figure 37B

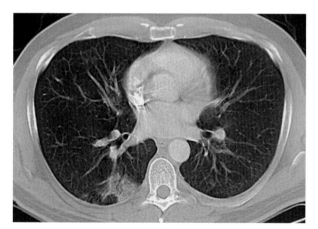

Figure 37C

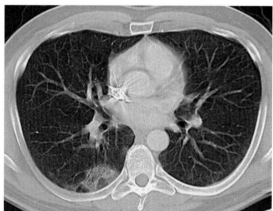

Figure 37D

Findings: PA and lateral chest radiographs showed a subtle, ill-defined right perihilar density. CT showed a similarly ill-defined parenchymal area of ground-glass opacity in the right lower lobe superior segment, with air bronchograms noted centrally within the lesion. There was also thickening around the right lower lobe bronchus.

Differential Diagnosis: BAC should be considered. A focal area of pneumonia would probably be the most likely diagnosis. For this reason the patient was given a trial of antibiotic therapy, with a repeat CT performed 2 weeks later. The area of concern persisted on the follow-up CT, prompting further evaluation with bronchoscopy and transbronchial biopsy.

Diagnosis: BAC.

Discussion: This is another example of BAC. Unlike the previous example, this lesion presented as a focal area of ground-glass opacity. However, a solitary, peripheral nodule is the most common presenting appearance of BAC. About half of patients are asymptomatic, as in this example, but cough, dyspnea, weight loss, and hemoptysis are possible symptoms. Bronchorrhea is the classic finding, but this is a late symptom seen in only 6% of patients.

High-resolution CT of BAC shows a peripheral, often spiculated nodule or a localized ground-glass attenuation with or without consolidation. Bubble-like lucencies representing patent bronchi are common.

Bronchioloalveolar carcinoma is believed to be the only malignancy that can spread along airways, giving a bronchopneumonia-type appearance. Lymphangitic carcinomatosis is also possible, resulting in an interstitial pattern on imaging studies.

Bronchioloalveolar carcinoma is thought to be more indolent than other adenocarcinomas. As compared with other bronchogenic adenocarcinomas matched for stage, better survival has been demonstrated for solitary lesions with and without ipsilateral hilar lymph node involvement. Size is an important prognostic factor, and lesions of less than 3 cm do very well.

SUGGESTED READING

Alasay K, Muller N, Ostrow DN, et al. Cryptogenic organizing pneumonia. A report of 25 cases and a review of the literature. *Medicine* 1995;74;201–211.

Aouad M, Berzina CE, Baraka AS. Aspiration pneumonia after anesthesia in a patient with Zenker diverticulum. *Anesthesiology* 2000;92: 1837–1839.

Barkley JE. Bronchioloalveolar carcinoma. *J Clin Oncol* 1996;14:2377–2386.

Barkley JE, Green MR. Bronchioloalveolar carcinoma. *J Clin Oncol* 1996;14:2377–2386.

Benditt JO, Farber HW, Wright J, et al. Pulmonary hemorrhage with diffuse alveolar infiltrates in men with high-volume choriocarcinoma. *Ann Intern Med* 1988;109:674–675.

Bhatt GM, Austin HM. CT demonstration of empyema necessitatis. *J Comput Assist Tomogr* 1985;9:1108–1109.

Bida MN, Mohlala ML. The right middle lobe syndrome—a case report and review of the literature. *S Afr Med J* 1997;87:178–179.

Billing DM, Darling DB. Middle lobe atelectasis in children: clinical and bronchographic criteria in the selection of patients for surgery. *Am J Dis Child* 1972;123:96–98.

Boiron P, Provost F, Chevrier G, et al. Review of nocardial infections in France 1987–1990. *Eur J Clin Microbiol Infect Dis* 1992;11:709–714.

Bouchardy LM, Kuhlman JE, Ball WC, et al. CT findings in bronchiolitis obliterans organizing pneumonia (BOOP) with radiographic, clinical, and histologic correlation. *J Comput Assist Tomogr* 1993;17:352–357.

Brock RC. Post-tuberculous broncho-stenosis and bronchiectasis of the middle lobe. *Thorax* 1950;5:5–39, 1950.

Buff SJ, McLelland R, Gallis HA, et al. *Candida albicans* pneumonia: radiographic appearance. *AJR Am J Roentgenol* 1982;138:645–648.

Byrd JC, Hargis JB, Kester KE, et al. Opportunistic pulmonary infections with fludarabine in previously treated patients with low grade lymphoid malignancies: a role for *Pneumocystis carinii* pneumonia prophylaxis. *Am J Hematol* 1995;49:135–142.

Carrigan A. Adenovirus infections in immunocompromised patients. *Am J Med* 1997;102:71–74.

Casey KR, Winterbauer RH. Persistent pulmonary infiltrate and bronchorrhea in a young woman. *Chest* 1997;111:1442–1445.

Cunha BA. Severe community acquired pneumonia. *Crit Care Clin* 1995;14:105–118.

Dalen JE, Haffajee CI, Alpert JS, et al. Pulmonary embolism, pulmonary hemorrhage and pulmonary infarction. *N Engl J Med* 1977;296: 1431–1435.

De Boeck K, Willems T, Van Gysel D, et al. Outcome after right middle lobe syndrome. *Chest* 1995;108:150–152.

Degregorio MW, Lee WMF, Linker CA, et al. Fungal infections in patients with acute leukemia. *Am J Med* 1982;73:543–548.

Dershaw DD. Actinomycosis of the chest wall: ultrasound findings in empyema necessitans. *Chest* 1984;86:779–780.

Epler GR. Heterogeneity of bronchiolitis obliterans organizing pneumonia. *Curr Opin Pulm Med* 1998;4:93–97.

Felson LB, Rosenberg LS, Hamburger M. Roentgen findings in acute Friedlander's pneumonia. *Radiology* 1949;53:559–565.

Georghiou PR, Blacklock ZM. Infection with *Nocardia* species in Queensland: a review of 102 clinical isolates. *Med J Aust* 1992;156: 692–697.

Gold R, Wilt JC, Adhikari PK, et al. Adenoviral pneumonia and its complications in infants and childhood. *J Can Assoc Radiol* 1969;20:218–224.

Goldstein LS, Kavuru MS, Curtis-McCarthy P, et al. Pulmonary alveolar proteinosis: clinical features and outcomes. *Chest* 1998;114: 1357–1362.

Haddad CJ, Sim WK. Empyema necessitatis. *Am Fam Physician* 1989;40:149–152.

Hamper UM, Fishman EK, Khouri NF, et al. Typical and atypical manifestations of pulmonary sarcoidosis. *J Comput Assist Tomogr* 1986; 10:925–935.

Hampton AO, Castleman B. Correlations of post-mortem chest teleroentgenograms with autopsy findings with special reference to pulmonary embolism and infarction. *AJR Am J Roentgenol* 1940;43:305–326.

Hansel DM, Kerr IH. The role of high resolution CT in the diagnosis of interstitial lung disease. *Thorax* 1991;46:77–84.

Herman PG, Khan A, Kallman CE. Limited correlation of left ventricular end-diastolic pressure with radiographic assessment of pulmonary hemodynamics. *Radiology* 1990;174:721–724.

Hierholzer JC. Adenoviruses in the immunocompromised host. *Clin Microbiol Rev* 1992;5:262–274.

Hockensmith ML, Mellman DL, Aronsen EL. Fusobacterium nucleatum empyema necessitans. *Clin Infect Dis* 1999;29:1596–1598.

Holmes RB. Friedlander's pneumonia. *AJR Am J Roentgenol* 1956;75:728–747.

Hsu CP, Chen CY, Hsu NY. Bronchioloalveolar carcinoma. *J Thorac Cardiovasc Surg* 1995;110:374–381.

Inner CR, Terry PB, Traytsman RS, et al. Collateral ventilation and the middle lobe syndrome. *Am Rev Respir Dis* 1978;118:305–310.

Jong GM, Hsiue TR, Chen CR, et al. Rapidly fatal outcome of bacteremic *Klebsiella* pneumonia in alcoholics. *Chest* 1995;107:214–217.

Katz DS, Leung AN. Radiology of pneumonia. *Clin Chest Med* 1999;20:549–562.

Kumar J, Ilancheran A, Ratnam SS. Pulmonary metastases in gestational trophoblastic disease: a review of 97 cases. *Br J Obstet Gynecol* 1988;95:70–74.

Landay MJ, Christensen EE, Bynum LJ. Pulmonary manifestations of acute aspiration of gastric contents. *AJR Am J Roentgenol* 1978;131: 587–592.

Lee K, Levin DL, Webb WR, et al. High-resolution CT, chest radiographic, and functional correlations. *Chest* 1997;111:989–995.

Lee KS, Hwang JW, Chung MP, et al. Utility of CT in the evaluation of pulmonary tuberculosis in patients without AIDS. *Chest* 1996;110: 997–984.

Lee KS, Kim Y, Han J, et al. Bronchioloalveolar carcinoma: clinical, histopathologic, and radiologic findings. *Radiographics* 1997;17: 1345–1357.

Leung AN, Muller N, Pinea PR, et al. Primary tuberculosis in childhood: radiographic manifestations, *Radiology* 1992;182:87–91.

Llibre JM, Urban A, Garcia E, et al. Bronchiolitis obliterans organizing pneumonia associated with acute *Mycoplasma pneumoniae* infection. *Clin Infect Dis* 1997;25:1340–1342.

Lohr RH, Boland BJ, Douglas WW, et al. Organizing pneumonia: features and prognosis of cryptogenic, secondary, and focal variants. *Arch Intern Med* 1997;157:1323–1329.

Mansharamani NG, Garland R, Delaney D, et al. Management and outcome patterns for adult *Pneumocystis carinii* pneumonia, 1985–1995: comparison of HIV-associated cases to other immunocompromised states. *Chest* 2000;118:704–711.

Marinella MA, Harrington GD, Standiford TJ. Empyema necessitans due to *Streptococcus milleri*. *Clin Infect Dis* 1996;23:203–204.

Marrie JJ. Community acquired pneumonia: epidemiology, etiology, and treatment. *Infect Dis Clin North Am* 1998;12:723–740.

Matthay MA. Pathophysiology of pulmonary edema. *Clin Chest Med* 1985;6:301–314.

Mazur MT, Lurain JF, Brewer JI. Fatal gestational choriocarcinoma. *Cancer* 1982;50:1833–1846.

McGowan MP, Pratter MR, Nash G. Primary testicular choriocarcinoma with pulmonary metastases presenting as ARDS. *Chest* 1990;97:1258–1259.

McHugh TJ, Forrester JS, Adler L, et al. Pulmonary vascular congestion in acute myocardial infarction: hemodynamic and radiologic correlations. *Ann Intern Med* 1972;76:29–33.

Menendez R, Cordero PJ, Santos M, et al. Pulmonary infection with *Nocardia* species: a report of 10 cases and review. *Eur Respir J* 1997;10:1542–1546.

Moon WK, Im JG, Yeon KM, et al. Complications of *Klebsiella* pneumonia: CT evaluation. *J Comput Assist Tomogr* 1995;19:176–181.

Murray JF, Mills J. Pulmonary infectious complications of human immunodeficiency virus infection, part I. *Am Rev Respir Dis* 1990;141:1356–1372.

Murray JF, Mills J. Pulmonary infectious complications of human immunodeficiency virus infection, part II. *Am Rev Respir Dis* 1990;141:1582–1598.

Nyman RS, Brismar J, Hugosson C, et al. Imaging of tuberculosis—experience from 503 patients. 1. Tuberculosis of the chest. *Acta Radiol* 1996;37:482–488.

Pagani JJ, Libshitz HI. Opportunistic fungal pneumonias in cancer patients. *AJR Am J Roentgenol* 1981;137:1033–1039.

Pistolesi M, Miniati M, Milne ENC, et al. The chest roentgenogram in pulmonary edema. *Clin Chest Med* 1985;6:315–344.

Provost F, Laurent F, Blanc MV, et al. Transmission of nocardiosis and molecular typing of *Nocardia* species: a short review. *Eur J Epidemiol* 1997;13:235–238.

Remy-Jardin M, Giraud F, Remy J, et al. Pulmonary sarcoidosis: role of CT in the evaluation of disease activity and functional impairment and in prognosis assessment. *Radiology* 1994;191:675–680.

Sindel EA. Empyema necessitatis. *Bull Sea View Hospital* 1940;6:1–49.

Skerret SJ. Diagnostic testing for community acquired pneumonia. *Clin Chest Med* 1999;20:531–548.

Sokolve PE. Implementation of an emergency department triage procedure for detection and isolation of patients with active pulmonary tuberculosis. *Ann Emerg Med* 2000;35:327–336.

Speckman DG, Spiteri MA. Sarcoidosis. *Postgrad Med J* 1996;72:196–200.

Springer C, Avital A, Noviski N, et al. Role of infection in the middle lobe syndrome in asthma. *Arch Dis Child* 1992;67:592–594.

Storto ML, Kee ST, Golden JA, et al. Hydrostatic pulmonary edema: high resolution CT findings. *AJR Am J Roentgenol* 1995;4:817–820.

Strand OA, Von der Lippe B, Stromsheim J. *Pneumocystis carinii* pneumonia—not only in AIDS. *Tidsskr Nor Laegeforen* 1992;112:2841–2842.

Tazi A. Pulmonary sarcoidosis with diffuse ground-glass pattern on chest radiograph. *Thorax* 1994;49:793–797.

Trak DM, Parkman HP, Fisher RS. Dysphagia: evaluation, diagnosis, and treatment. *Prim Care* 1996;23:417–432.

Vix VA. The usefulness of chest radiographs obtained after a demonstrated perfusion scan defect in the diagnosis of pulmonary emboli. *Clin Nucl Med* 1983;8:497–500.

Vogeser M, Wanders A, Haas A, et al. A four-year review of fatal aspergillosis. *Eur J Clin Microbiol Infect Dis* 1999;18:42–45.

Walker PA, White DA. Management of the HIV-infected patient. Part 1: Pulmonary disease. *Med Clin North Am* 1996;80:1337–1362.

Wang BM, Stern EJ, Schmidt RA, et al. Diagnosing pulmonary alveolar proteinosis: a review and update. *Chest* 1997;111:460–466.

Watemberg S, Landau O, Avraham R. Zenker's diverticulum: reappraisal. *Am J Gastroenterol* 1996;91:1494–1498.

Zahhradnik JM. Adenovirus pneumonia. *Semin Respir Infect* 1987;2:104–111.

Zapatero J, Bellon J, Baamondi C, et al. Primary choriocarcinoma of the lung: presentation of a case and review of the literature. *Scand J Thorac Cardiovasc Surg* 1982;16:279–281.

CHAPTER 3

INTERSTITIAL LUNG DISEASE

RUNI A. FOSTER
PATRICIA J. MERGO

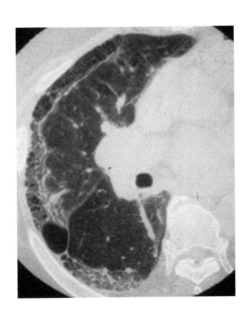

CASE 38

History: A 52-year-old man with a previous history of lung cancer presented with increasing shortness of breath.

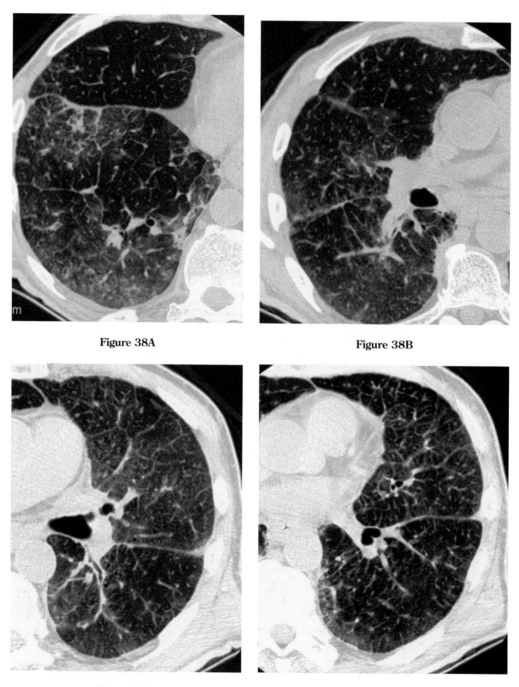

Figure 38A

Figure 38B

Figure 38C

Figure 38D

Findings: Helical CT and HRCT were performed. The HRCT images showed predominantly a central peribronchial interstitial disease, although there was some peripheral interstitial thickening of the intralobular septa. There were scattered ground-glass changes in the dependent portions of the lung, both in the upper and lower lobes.

Diagnosis: Pulmonary edema, HRCT findings.

Discussion: HRCT showed ground-glass attenuation of the lungs. This is a nonspecific finding seen with many entities. One common cause of ground-glass changes within the lungs is pulmonary edema, as seen in this case. In addition, there was interstitial edema with thickening of the intralobular septa in the periphery of the lungs, as well as central peribronchial interstitial thickening. At the time of the patient's presentation, there was concern that there may have been lymphangitic spread of his previously detected lung cancer. His clinical course and history was not consistent with the presentation of lymphangitic spread of carcinoma, and this was not confirmed on histologic examination. However, the histologic changes and clinical course were consistent with those of transient pulmonary edema related to congestive failure. Enlargement of the pulmonary veins at the lung bases was evident, which also correlates with pulmonary venous vascular congestion.

CASE 39

History: A 70-year-old ex-smoker with a history of silicosis presented with 250 mL of hemoptysis over the preceding 24 hours. Prior to admission, he reported having intermittent blood-streaked sputum for the preceding 6 months. He also admitted to a 23-pound weight loss with increasing dyspnea but denied having fevers, night sweats, or chills.

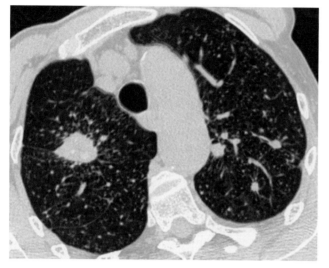

Figure 39A

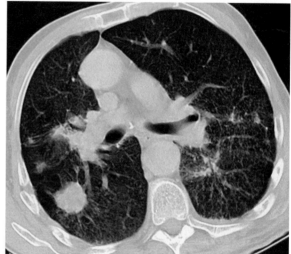

Figure 39B

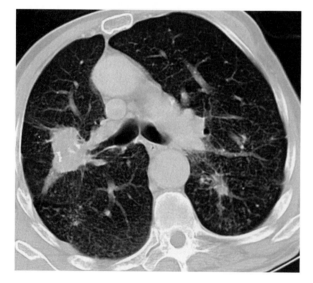

Figure 39C

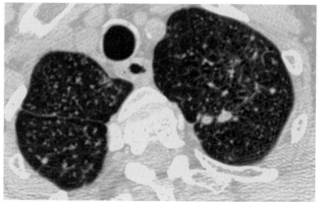

Figure 39D

Findings: Lung windows demonstrated a reticular nodular interstitial pattern. Although there was some peripheral interstitial changes, with thickening of the intralobular septa, the pattern was that of a predominantly central peribronchial interstitial process. There were more conglomerate areas of masslike consolidation evident, which contained calcifications as well.

Differential Diagnosis: Metastatic carcinoma or bronchogenic carcinoma can present with symptoms of hemoptysis along with weight loss. Another entity that should be considered in the differential diagnosis is reactivation TB, because of the increased incidence of *Mycobacterium tuberculosis* in this patient population.

Diagnosis: Silicosis with PMF.

Discussion: Because this illness is rare, silicosis is often misdiagnosed. Radiographic abnormalities are noted before clinical presentation. The diagnosis is made with a thorough occupational history. Radiographically, silicotic lung disease appears very similar to coal worker's pneumoconiosis.

This patient was a coal miner with significant exposure to silica dust. The findings were typical of silicosis, with central lobular peribronchial interstitial thickening. There was associated intralobular septal thickening as well. Central lobular interstitial thickening can be seen with several disease entities, including silicosis, pulmonary edema, sarcoidosis, and lymphangitic spread of carcinoma. Interstitial nodules can be seen with granulomatous processes, such as sarcoidosis, histiocytosis X, silicosis, and coal worker's pneumoconiosis, as well as TB, lymphangitic spread of tumor, and hypersensitivity pneumonia. Several images showed subpleural interstitial nodules in the upper lobes, typical of coal worker's pneumoconiosis and silicosis. This case nicely demonstrates a finding of more conglomerate masses, which are known as PMF. These masses are conglomerate aggregates of granulomatous change that coalesce with the changes of fibrosis and longstanding disease. These conglomerate fibrotic changes result in architectural distortion and retraction of the hila upward.

Chronic silicosis is the most common manifestation of silicotic lung disease. It is caused by chronic low-level exposure to crystallized silicon dioxide. The type of presentation is dependent on the length of exposure. Individuals who inhale a significant quantity of silicotic dust can develop rapid progressive nodular changes with associated massive fibrosis, whereas patients with chronic low-level exposure develop more indolent nodular radiographic abnormalities.

The earliest manifestation of silicosis is nodular densities, which measure a few millimeters in diameter and are predominantly seen in the upper lobes and perihilar regions. CT and HRCT are superior to chest radiography in localizing small upper lobe nodules. The appearance of larger nodules, also known as conglomerate masses or PMF, indicates the presence of complicated silicosis. PMF on CT appears as a masslike consolidation with associated apical parenchymal scarring and adjacent bullous emphysema. Calcification within the masses is common. Coal worker's pneumoconiosis can present with similar CT findings, but the masses are oval in shape with irregular borders and fewer incidences of emphysematous changes. In masses that are larger than 4 cm, there are usually areas of central necrosis with cavitation.

Tuberculosis and pneumothorax can complicate silicosis, with rupture of bullae causing the pleural air. Cavitation from TB can be difficult to differentiate from underlying lung disease, but mycobacterial disease should be suspected if there has been a rapid change in the cavities. Tuberculous cavities, superimposed bacterial infections, or broncholithiasis can cause significant hemoptysis. Diagnosis is made clinically by the new onset of systemic symptoms, along with cultures and possibly bronchoscopy.

CASE 40

History: This patient was a 60-year-old woman with a 25-year history of sarcoidosis. She was oxygen dependent and had produced less than a cup of hemoptysis daily in the preceding 48 hours.

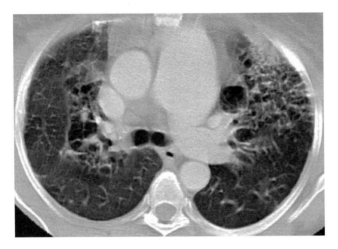

Figure 40A

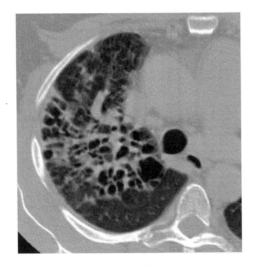

Figure 40B

Findings: CT on the day of admission showed prominent cystic changes from end-stage honeycombing throughout both lungs. Bronchiectatic changes were superimposed on the cystic changes. In addition, the central pulmonary artery was markedly enlarged from secondary changes of pulmonary hypertension from the patient's underlying lung disease.

Differential Diagnosis: Bilateral cystic changes with bronchiectasis in patients with end-stage sarcoidosis can represent superimposed opportunistic infections such as *Mycobacterium* species or fungal infections such as chronic cavitary aspergillosis.

Diagnosis: End-stage lung disease with pulmonary hypertension from sarcoidosis.

Discussion: Sarcoidosis is staged based on chest radiographic findings which have been useful in assessing prognosis and guiding in therapeutic options. The classification is as follows: stage 0, normal chest radiograph; stage I, BHL without infiltrates; stage II, BHL plus infiltrates; stage III, pulmonary infiltrates without BHL; stage IV (not universally adopted), extensive fibrosis with distortion, cavitation, and bullae formation.

The clinical presentation of sarcoidosis is vast, but the majority of patients have pulmonary symptoms. Almost all patients with sarcoidosis have radiographic abnormalities. Chronic pulmonary sarcoidosis such as stage IV is associated with reduced lung function, progressive dyspnea, and hypoxemia, with eventual chronic respiratory failure and death.

High-resolution CT is superior to conventional CT in showing parenchymal detail and differentiating alveolitis from fibrosis. CT and HRCT in stage IV sarcoidosis demonstrate architectural distortion, septal thickening, enlarged pulmonary arteries, traction bronchiectasis, and honeycombing with cystic destruction. CT abnormalities can guide therapy, especially for those patients who have ground-glass appearance, which suggests alveolitis, whereas those with fibrosis may benefit more from conservative management.

Complications from this lung disease include stenosis or compression of bronchi from inflammation, or extrinsic compression from the lymph nodes and pulmonary hypertension, as seen in this patient. CT scans are useful in determining the extent of stenosis in the lower respiratory tract. Aspergillomas, which occur in 10% of patients, may be a life-threatening complication; they develop in the cystic spaces with stage III or IV sarcoidosis.

Treatment options for stage IV sarcoidosis are limited, with poor response unless there is evidence of alveolitis on the CT scan.

CASE 41

History: A 65-year-old man with a history of a chronic lung disease presented with a chronic cough of several months' duration.

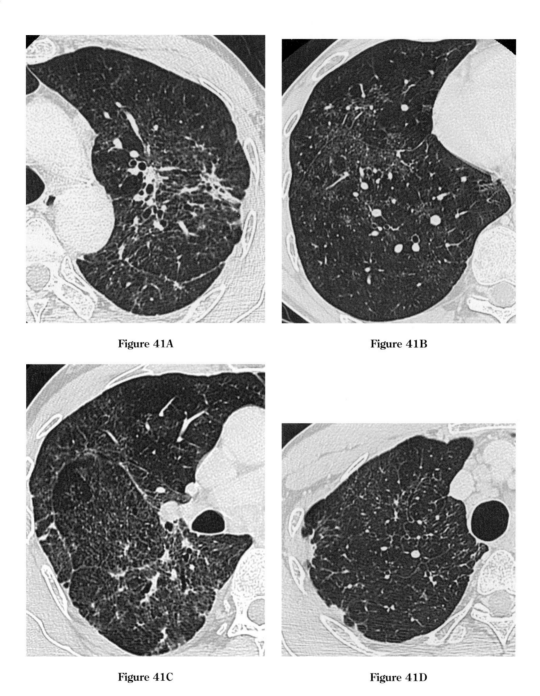

Figure 41A

Figure 41B

Figure 41C

Figure 41D

Findings: The patient's lung parenchyma showed evidence of interstitial lung disease, with a miliary nodular component in the right middle lung zones bilaterally. No evidence for associated pleural effusion was identified, although there was some pleural thickening. No enlarged hilar adenopathy was identified. The patient's central pulmonary vasculature did not appear to be enlarged.

Differential Diagnosis: In a patient with a new onset of cough and miliary pattern on the radiograph, one must suspect TB, hypersensitivity pneumonitis, and lymphangitic carcinomatosis. If the patient has any applicable occupational history, pneumoconiosis (such as silicosis or asbestosis) also should be considered.

Diagnosis: Stage III sarcoidosis.

Discussion: When patients develop chronic sarcoidosis, only 50% of them are asymptomatic; the remainder have systemic symptoms such as fever, weight loss, night sweats, dry cough, and dyspnea, with a minority of patients developing hemoptysis. Cough or dyspnea may be the prominent symptoms in patients with endobronchial or parenchymal sarcoidosis, as in this patient.

Stage III sarcoidosis occurs in approximately 15% to 20% of patients with pulmonary sarcoidosis, with spontaneous remission occurring in only 10% to 20% of patients with this stage of disease.

High-resolution CT may be superior to conventional CT in defining the parenchymal abnormalities, such as alveolitis versus fibrotic lung disease. Conventional CT may be preferable for identifying miliary and peribronchovascular nodules. Characteristic findings in stage III sarcoidosis include (a) smooth, well-defined nodules and micronodules that are less than 3 mm in diameter along the bronchovascular bundles, (b) peribronchial interstitial thickening, (c) central distribution with eventual involvement of the upper lobes and apical scarring, and (d) ground-glass opacities suggesting active alveolitis.

CASE 42

History: A 26-year-old man who was previously healthy presented with a progressively worsening cough and dyspnea on exertion.

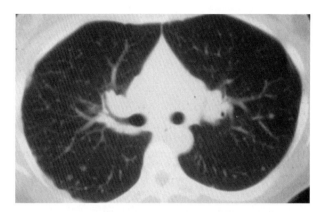

Figure 42A

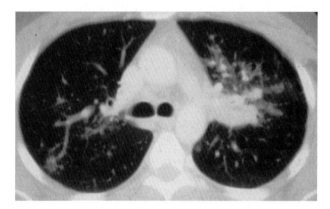

Figure 42B

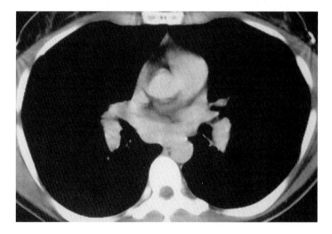

Figure 42C

Findings: Lung windows and mediastinal windows from contrast-enhanced CT of the chest showed central peribronchial interstitial thickening and nodularity emanating from both hilar regions. Multiple small nodules were also evident in the lung parenchyma, as was bilateral hilar adenopathy.

Diagnosis: Sarcoidosis.

Discussion: This case nicely illustrates the pattern of interstitial involvement of the lungs from sarcoidosis with central peribronchial interstitial thickening. The peribronchial soft tissues were markedly thickened all the way to the hilar regions with more peripheral parenchymal nodularity evident. Given this patient's age and history, sarcoidosis is a likely diagnosis, but lymphoma is also a primary diagnostic consideration. Bronchoscopy was performed and the results of transbronchial biopsy showed noncaseating granulomas consistent with sarcoidosis. Silicosis and lymphangitic carcinomatosis also can have this pattern of involvement of the central peribronchial interstitium.

The distribution of sarcoidosis seen on CT is compatible with lung biopsy findings, in which the noncaseating granulomas are more commonly seen in the bronchovascular region than in the subpleural region. Sarcoidosis and lymphangitic carcinomatosis have similar bronchovascular distribution, whereas IPF is commonly seen in the peripheral and lower lung region. With progression of this disease, patients develop traction bronchiectasis, fibrosis, cavitation, and conglomerate masses.

CASE 43

History: A 29-year-old woman presented with worsening severe dyspnea and a nonproductive cough. She was a non-smoker and had no prior history of lung disease.

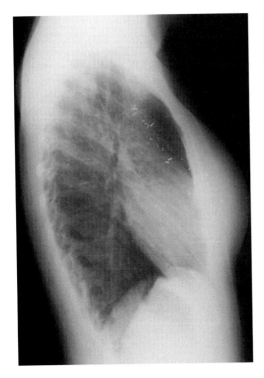

Figure 43A

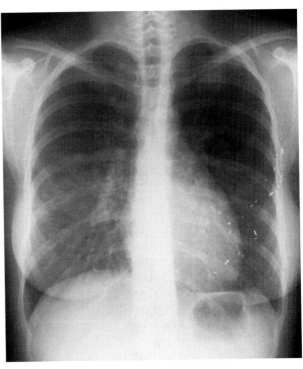

Figure 43B

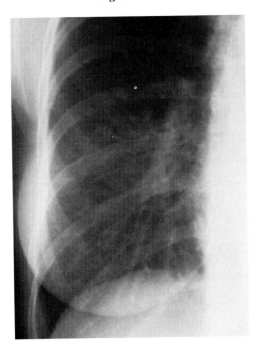

Figure 43C

Findings: PA and lateral chest radiographs and a cone-down view of the right lower lung fields showed a diffuse nodular interstitial pattern in the lungs. Extensive surgical clips were seen overlying the left chest, with some asymmetry evident in the overlying breast tissue.

Diagnosis: Lymphangitic carcinomatosis from breast cancer.

Discussion: Lymphangitic spread of lung cancer or lymphangitic carcinomatosis results from tumor cells invading the lymphatics, which causes lymphatic vessel dilatation, surrounding interstitial edema, and a degree of thickening or fibrosis.

The radiologic pattern associated with lymphangitic spread of tumor is a nodular or smooth thickening of the interlobular septa and peribronchovascular interstitium, which does not distort the pulmonary lobule. The interlobular septa are thickened out to the peripheral 1 cm of the lung, where their thickened appearance is often initially recognized. Interstitial nodular thickening can be seen as well. The underlying lung architecture is usually preserved, however. When this pattern is seen in a patient without a known primary malignancy, transbronchial biopsy is often helpful in making the diagnosis. Lung cancer is a common cause of lymphangitic carcinomatosis and can present as a unilateral process. Extrapulmonary neoplasms that commonly result in lymphangitic carcinomatosis include those of the breast, stomach, pancreas, colon, prostate, and cervix, which typically cause a more usual bilateral appearance.

CASE 44

History: A 53-year-old woman underwent malignant melanoma resection of the thigh 8 years prior to presentation and subsequently had resection of a metastatic lesion in the right ulna. Two weeks later she presented with increasing dyspnea, cough, and blood-streaked sputum.

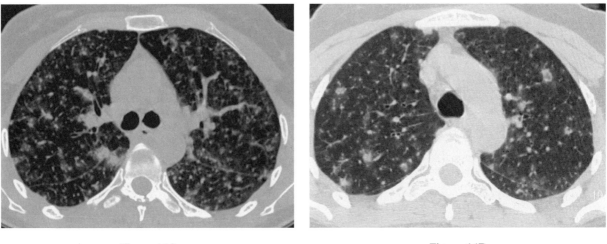

Figure 44A   Figure 44B

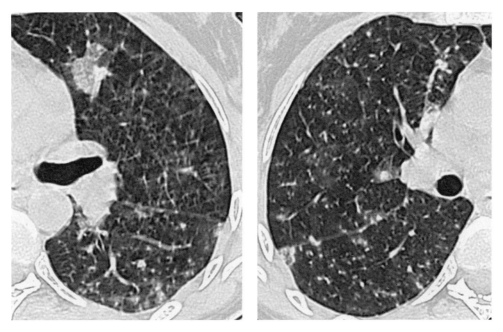

Figure 44C   Figure 44D

Findings: A diffuse, coarsely nodular interstitial pattern was present bilaterally, involving both the upper and lower lung zones. There were areas of more confluent nodularity, with the largest of these areas in the region of the left upper lobe measuring approximately 2×2 cm. Multiple smaller nodules were identified. All of the nodular areas had rather ill-defined borders.

Differential Diagnosis: A variety of disorders can manifest with similar symptoms; extrinsic allergic alveolitis can present with a similar radiographic pattern, but large nodular masses are seldom seen with allergic alveolitis. Other entities include sarcoidosis, which can imitate other disease processes and may have similar HRCT findings. A final entity that should be considered is IPF in the early fibrotic phase of the disease process.

Diagnosis: Lymphangitic carcinomatosis.

Discussion: Lymphangitic carcinomatosis occurs in approximately 7% of all metastatic carcinomas to the lung. It occurs by tumor embolization of the blood vessels with subsequent lymphatic obstruction, edema, and eventual deposition of tumor cells within the lymphatic system. Lymphangitic spread occurs most frequently in adenocarcinomas; thus, it is mostly seen with breast, bronchogenic, stomach, cervix, pancreas, colon, and thyroid carcinomas, and occasionally metastatic adenocarcinoma of unknown origin.

The symptoms always predate the radiographic findings and usually include insidious onset of dyspnea, dry cough, and weight loss. Patients occasionally have hemoptysis as a presenting symptom.

Chest radiographs are nonspecific but reveal patchy, reticular opacities with thickened septal lines and small lung volumes, and occasionally can appear to be normal. HRCT has characteristic findings, including reticular opacities with a nodular appearance. Specific abnormalities include smooth or nodular peribronchial thickening of the interlobular septa, axial interstitial thickening [which can also have a smooth or nodular (beaded) pattern], no architectural distortion of the lung, and evidence of small lung volumes. These findings are observed in approximately 50% of the patients.

The thickened septal lines are approximately 1 to 2 cm in length and have contact with the pleural space; the beaded appearance seen in the interstitium is a result of tumor growth within the interstitium, capillaries, and the lymphatics. The lung architecture is maintained with the appearance of normal pulmonary lobules, whereas another diagnosis should be considered if there is loss of normal pulmonary architecture or lobular distortion.

CASE 45

History: A 26-year-old woman with a history of Hodgkin's disease treated multiple times for recurrence presented with fevers and night sweats, and was completing a course of antibiotics and steroid therapy.

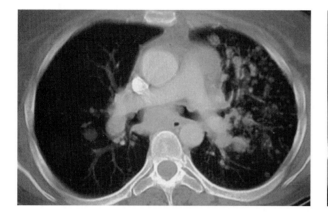

Figure 45A

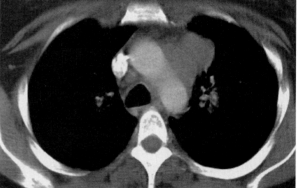

Figure 45B

Findings: CT of the chest with contrast demonstrated extensive mediastinal adenopathy in the aorticopulmonary window and prevascular space. The largest conglomerate group of nodes in the prevascular space measured 4.5 cm. Examination of the lung parenchyma demonstrated innumerable small nodules in the left lung parenchyma, ranging in size from 5 mm to 2 cm. These nodules coursed along the central peribronchial interstitium and were most concentrated in the upper lobe. A few scattered subcentimeter nodules were present in the right lung as well.

Differential Diagnosis: This patient was immunocompromised and presented with fevers. Thus, one must be concerned about an opportunistic infection such as disseminated aspergillosis or nocardiosis, which can present as multiple pulmonary nodules on the radiograph. Sarcoidosis also may present in a similar fashion, but given this patient's history it is very unlikely the cause of her symptoms.

Diagnosis: Diffuse recurrent Hodgkin's disease.

Discussion: Forty percent of all lymphomas manifest as Hodgkin's disease. Upon presentation, approximately 65% of Hodgkin's disease cases manifest with intrathoracic disease, such as lymph node enlargement within the mediastinum or lymphoid aggregates within the bronchi or in the region of the parietal pleura. Nodular sclerosing Hodgkin's disease also can present with parenchymal abnormalities in 15% to 30% of patients. The most common type of involvement seen on CT includes a coarse reticulonodular pattern with direct extension from the mediastinum along the lymphatics. Parenchymal nodules of varying sizes also may be seen. Rarely patients present with atelectasis and lung collapse due to endobronchial involvement. Pleural effusion can be seen in 25% to 50% of cases due to pleural involvement of the lymphoma or from lymphatic obstruction. Other manifestations include diffuse nonsegmental or lobar infiltrates with evidence of air bronchograms or as subcentimeter pulmonary nodules, which is suggestive of metastatic disease.

Because the majority of these patients are immunocompromised, a diagnostic procedure such as bronchoscopy, CT-guided needle biopsy, or open lung biopsy should be performed to exclude an opportunistic infection.

CASE 46

History: A 52-year-old man with a history of weight loss, fevers, and a mildly productive cough.

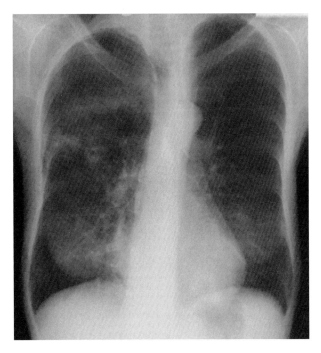

Figure 46

Findings: A PA radiographic view of the chest showed hyperinflation of the lungs with central peribronchial interstitial thickening and nodularity. There was also a more confluent area of airspace opacity in the right upper lobe.

Differential Diagnosis: Diagnostic considerations should include lymphangitic carcinomatosis, silicosis, sarcoidosis, fungal infection, and TB, and less likely lymphoma.

Diagnosis: *Mycobacterium tuberculosis* infection.

Discussion: This case demonstrates another example of abnormal thickening of the central peribronchial interstitium, in this instance caused by infection with TB. Interstitial nodular thickening was evident in this case, although the classic miliary pattern of nodules 2 to 3 mm in diameter was not evident.

Reactivation TB has a classic predilection for the posterior aspects of the upper lobes and the superior segments of the lower lobes. The airspace pattern seen in reactivation begins with a patchy consolidation with indistinct margins that may spread to involve the entire lobe. Cavitation and pleural effusion are common accompanying features. The disease spreads throughout the lungs via the airway, creating a bronchoalveolar pattern of small, patchy infiltrates bilaterally.

CASE 47

History: A 78-year-old man with a 3-year history of increasing dyspnea and a 1-year history of nonproductive cough. The patient was dependent on supplemental oxygen therapy.

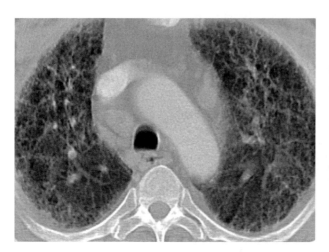

Figure 47A

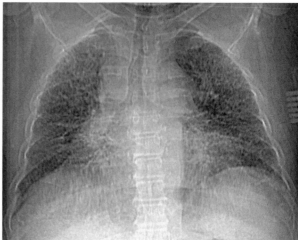

Figure 47B

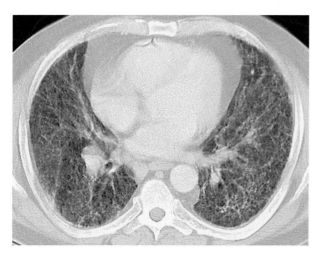

Figure 47C

Findings: A scout topographic image showed decreased lung volumes with increased interstitial markings. HRCT examination demonstrated marked interstitial thickening, predominantly in the lung bases with subpleural blebs present bilaterally, also primarily in the lung bases. Interstitial interlobular septal thickening was most marked in the periphery of the lung.

Differential Diagnosis: CT results and the patient's history are suggestive of chronic lung disease; therefore, etiologies such as rheumatoid lung, scleroderma, asbestosis, or fibrosing alveolitis should be considered.

Diagnosis: IPF or cryptogenic fibrosing alveolitis.

Discussion: IPF, also known as cryptogenic fibrosing alveolitis, is a chronic interstitial lung disease of unknown etiology. The classification of IPF has undergone several revisions and now is described as four histologic types: (a) usual interstitial pneumonia (UIP), (b) desquamative interstitial pneumonia (DIP), (c) acute interstitial pneumonitis (AIP), and (d) nonspecific interstitial pneumonitis (NSIP). UIP is the most common subtype, with insidious onset, poor response to steroids, and a 5-year mortality rate of greater than 50%.

High-resolution CT is being used increasingly to detect early forms of IPF when plain films have been equivocal or normal to prevent delay in treatment and progression of further lung damage. HRCT can provide information such as prognosis, extent, and pattern of the disease. HRCT manifestations of IPF are dependent on the disease course, with ground-glass appearance suggestive of alveolitis; the alveolitis pattern is nonspecific and can be seen in any of the subtypes of IPF. The fibrotic pattern provides more information regarding prognosis. When there is greater than 25% fibrosis of the lungs, it is associated with the worst prognosis and a poor response to treatment.

High-resolution CT of IPF shows a reticulonodular pattern within the lung bases with a prominent reticular pattern as the disease progresses. The most characteristic finding in IPF is the predilection of the disease process to occur in the subpleural and lower lobe region. The earliest sign of IPF is faint subpleural opacification in the lower lobes. As the disease progresses, a reticular pattern is seen, with formation of small cystic air spaces within the periphery of the lung parenchyma. These cystic spaces eventually develop into a honeycomb pattern. Another notable feature of this disease is decreased lung volumes and the development of traction bronchiectasis due to the distortion of the bronchi from the scarred interstitium.

Overall, lung parenchymal findings are indistinguishable from those of asbestosis. HRCT shows thickening of the peripheral interlobular septa seen as short interstitial lines. Longer, thicker parenchymal bands generally extend out to the pleural surface and course over a distance of 2 to 5 cm, and subpleural lines extend along the subpleural lung surface. Eighty percent of patients with asbestosis show associated asbestos-related pleural thickening, helping to distinguish between the two entities.

CASE 48

History: A 30-year-old male smoker with recurrent pneumonia in the left lower lobe.

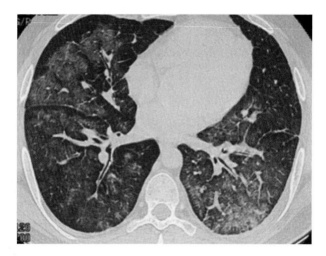

Figure 48

Findings: A single CT image of the chest showed diffuse ground-glass changes throughout all the lung fields, but most prominent in the lung bases. More focal airspace opacity and acinar filling were seen in the left lower lobe.

Differential Diagnosis: Etiologies of infiltrates in a young person could include inhalational injury, atypical pneumonia such as viral or *Pneumocystis* pneumonia, lupus pneumonitis, BOOP, hypersensitivity pneumonitis, or eosinophilic pneumonia.

Diagnosis: DIP.

Discussion: DIP is a distinct and separate clinical entity from UIP. DIP is seen in a younger population with insidious onset and has a more favorable prognosis compared with UIP. DIP has distinct pathologic features with an increased number of macrophages with abundant cytoplasm within the alveolar sacs. There is minimal to moderate septal widening. Fibroblast proliferation is not characteristic of DIP. The overall appearance on low magnification is that of a homogenous pattern of involvement, unlike the heterogeneous and patchy distribution seen in UIP.

The CT findings in DIP are diffuse ground-glass changes of the lungs with minimal interstitial thickening. Unlike UIP, there is a random distribution of the disease with no subpleural predilection and no evidence of honeycombing. Patients with DIP respond to steroids and can have complete resolution of their infiltrates.

CASE 49

History: A 33-year-old woman with a history of a chronic inflammatory condition presented with progressive shortness of breath. She had no history of fever, night sweats, or chills.

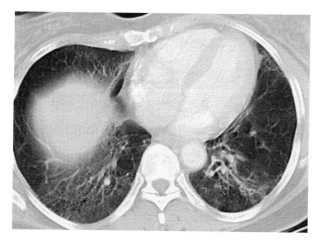

Figure 49A

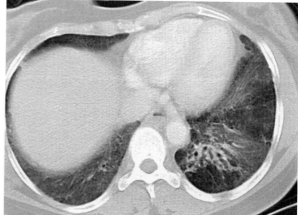

Figure 49B

Findings: Two images from CT of the chest in lung windows showed diffuse lower lobe interstitial changes with thickening of the interlobular septae in the periphery of the lung and mild associated bronchiectatic changes in the left lower lobe. Ground-glass changes were present in the lower lobes.

Diagnosis: Pulmonary involvement from systemic lupus erythematosus (SLE or lupus).

Discussion: Pulmonary involvement in lupus is not uncommon, with 50% to 70% of lupus patients having pleuropulmonary manifestations. Pleuritis and infection are the most common pulmonary manifestations of lupus. Bacterial or viral pneumonias are common and should be considered in any patient with lupus who presents with fever, cough, and shortness of breath. Parenchymal inflammation from pulmonary involvement of lupus itself is less common than pleural involvement, with approximately 5% of patients with lupus experiencing acute lupus pneumonitis. Fibrosing alveolitis as a result of lupus is even less common, occurring in less than 3% of lupus patients.

Overall, the most common pulmonary manifestation of lupus is pleural involvement, with either pleuritis or a pleural effusion. Pleuritis is seen in approximately 50% of patients with SLE. When an effusion is present, it is usually exudative in nature and may contain antinuclear antibodies. Pleural thickening also may be seen.

When present, the findings of fibrosing alveolitis are similar to those depicted in this case, with basilar peripheral interstitial changes evident with thickened interlobular septae noted on HRCT. Ground-glass changes also may be seen. Overall, the findings resemble those seen with IPF.

CASE 50

History: A 55-year-old man presented with progressive onset of worsening shortness of breath and a 2- to 3-year history of a nonproductive cough.

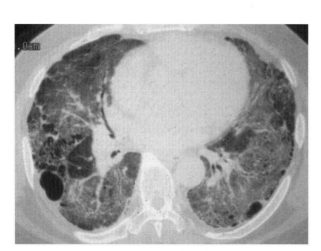

Figure 50A

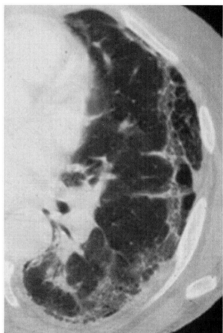

Figure 50B

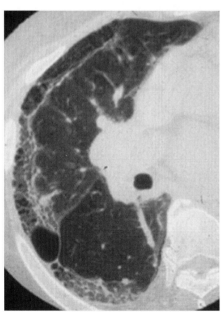

Figure 50C

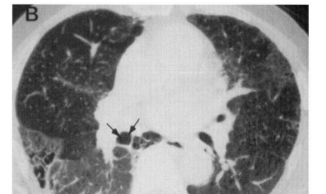

Figure 50D

Findings: Four HRCT images showed extensive subpleural cyst formation and thickening of the peripheral interlobular septae. Cone-down views of the left lower lobe and right lower lobe showed multiple subpleural lines, many of which were evident in the nondependent portion of the lung (as well as some in the dependent portion of the lung). Centrally, there was traction bronchiectasis *(arrows)*.

Diagnosis: Asbestosis.

Discussion: The findings in this case are classic for asbestosis, although the same findings can be seen with IPF.

Asbestos is composed of a group of minerals that are fibrous and resistant to high temperatures and chemical insults. They are divided into two major groups: curved fibers and straight fibers. There are three main sources of exposure: (a) primary exposure from asbestos mining and its processing in a mill; (b) secondary exposure from its use in industrial and commercial products such as construction, the automotive industry, and shipbuilding; and (c) airborne exposure of persons who are not in asbestos-related occupations.

Clinically, there is a latent period of 20 to 40 years between exposure and disease. The majority of patients are asymptomatic. They may have pleural pain associated with a pleural effusion. In the late stages, they may develop shortness of breath from interstitial fibrosis. On examination, these patients have crackles in the lung bases. This finding associated with a history of asbestos exposure is sufficient to make a diagnosis of asbestosis. Pulmonary function tests show a restrictive pattern.

Pulmonary asbestosis is the term reserved for diffuse parenchymal interstitial fibrosis, most commonly seen in the subpleural regions of the lower lobes. The lung changes occur in three stages. First, a fine reticulation pattern with associated ground-glass appearance is seen predominantly in the lower lung zones. Then the reticular pattern becomes more prominent. In the late stage, the reticulation is severe and may involve all lung zones. HRCT shows thickening of the peripheral interlobular septa, seen as short interstitial lines. Longer, thicker parenchymal bands generally extend out to the pleural surface and course over a distance of 2 to 5 cm, and subpleural lines extend along the subpleural lung surface. Approximately 80% of patients have pleural thickening and plaques. The finding of pleural involvement may help cement the diagnosis of asbestosis, because the interstitial parenchymal changes are otherwise indistinguishable from IPF.

CASE 51

History: A 59-year-old male ex-smoker with a 10-year history of a chronic inflammatory disease and associated shortness of breath.

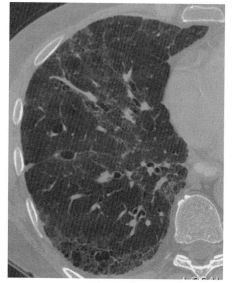

Figure 51A

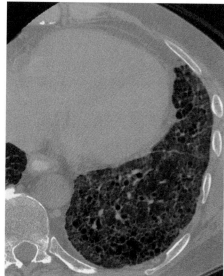

Figure 51B

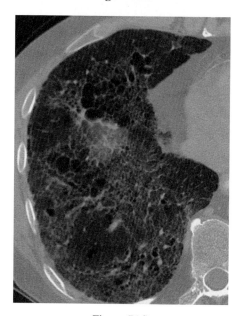

Figure 51C

Findings: Extensive coarse reticular interstitial disease was evident on HRCT, with subpleural cystic changes from honeycombing and associated traction bronchiectasis. The findings were bilateral, with the lung bases involved much more than the apices. A persistent contrast-filled mildly dilated esophagus was noted incidentally.

Differential Diagnosis: Due to the appearance of the thickened interstitium, chronic lung disease such as UIP, sarcoidosis, and rheumatoid or scleroderma lung should be considered in the differential diagnosis.

Diagnosis: Scleroderma.

Discussion: It was initially thought that interstitial lung disease only occurred in patients with scleroderma and not CREST syndrome. Now, it is known that interstitial lung disease occurs in both clinical entities. With progression of lung disease, scleroderma patients develop exertional dyspnea, but eventually they develop dyspnea at rest. As in other fibrotic chronic lung disease, signs of cor pulmonale eventually appear.

The initial sign of pulmonary disease on a plain film is usually a bibasilar interstitial pattern of disease. However, HRCT is much more sensitive in detecting early lung disease when the chest radiograph is normal. As the disease progresses, radiographic abnormalities include honeycombing, a decrease in lung volumes, and pulmonary vascular enlargement, suggesting pulmonary hypertension. Older data suggest that the 5-year survival rate for patients with interstitial lung disease is less than 50%. Recently, pathologic correlation of inflammatory cells in bronchoalveolar lavage along with ground-glass appearance on HRCT suggests that there is potential for response to steroids.

Other pulmonary manifestations of scleroderma include (a) pleural disease predominantly as pleural fibrosis rather than pleural effusions, (b) pulmonary hypertension more commonly seen in patients with CREST syndrome, (c) bronchiolitis obliterans, and (d) aspiration pneumonia.

CASE 52

History: A 41-year-old woman with a 17-year history of Raynaud's phenomenon, and shortness of breath of several months' duration.

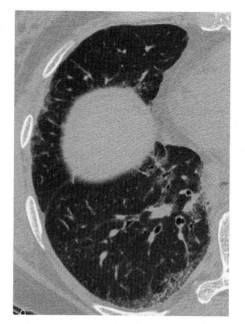

Figure 52A

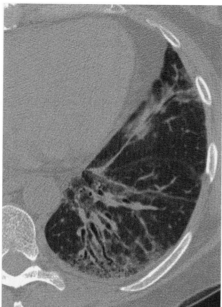

Figure 52B

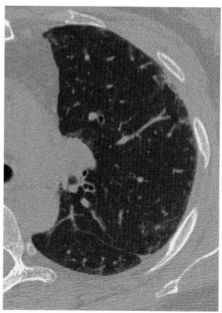

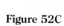

Figure 52C

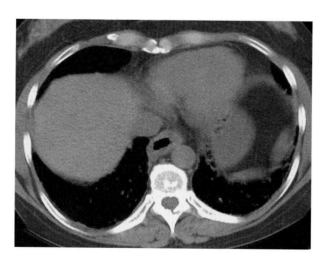

Figure 52D

Findings: The lung volumes were decreased. Bibasilar fibrotic changes were noted on HRCT, with peripheral interstitial thickening from thickening of the interlobular septa. The upper lobes were also involved, but to a lesser degree than the lower lobes. Associated mild traction bronchiectatic changes were noted in both lower lobes. There were also findings of secondary involvement of the esophagus, with a mildly dilated esophagus noted incidentally by CT.

Differential Diagnosis: The decreased lung volumes along with the fibrotic interstitial changes are consistent with chronic lung disease, such as UIP, rheumatoid lung, end-stage sarcoidosis, or scleroderma.

Diagnosis: Scleroderma.

Discussion: Scleroderma, also known as systemic sclerosis, is an inflammatory-fibrotic disorder of connective tissue that results in excessive deposition of fibrotic matrix within the vessels of the skin and internal organs. In autopsy series, pulmonary involvement was noted in 70% to 80% of cases. Scleroderma is three times more common in women than in men. Progressive dyspnea develops in these patients, but it is unusual for them to have this symptom at the time of initial presentation.

Computed tomography scans can show signs of early interstitial lung disease despite normal chest radiographs. Interstitial pneumonitis is the most common pulmonary manifestation of systemic sclerosis. Plain radiographs cannot be used to detect early lung disease from scleroderma because up to 44% of patients with normal radiographs can have an abnormal CT scan. HRCT in scleroderma has correlated with pathologic findings. Ground-glass opacification without traction bronchiectasis suggests active inflammation, whereas increased interstitial markings have correlated with fibrosis on pathologic specimens. The interstitial changes are nonspecific and are similar to those of rheumatoid lung disease, UIP, and mixed connective tissue disorders. The most common HRCT findings in scleroderma are subpleural lines in the dorsal region, honeycombing, parenchymal bands, thickened septa, and subpleural cysts.

Although HRCT is superior to plain radiographs in identifying the lung changes associated with this disease, the information obtained so far has not been applied for determination of therapeutic response and prognostic importance.

CASE 53

History: A 47-year-old man with a known history of chronic lymphocytic leukemia. He had undergone bone marrow transplantation, and presented with worsening dyspnea on exertion, a nonproductive cough, and decreased oxygen saturation. He had no history of fevers or chills.

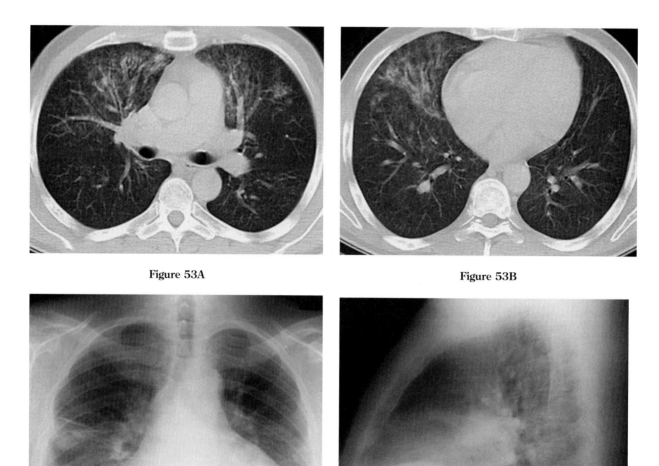

Figure 53A

Figure 53B

Figure 53C

Figure 53D

Findings: PA and lateral radiographic views of the chest showed decreased lung volumes with peripheral areas of consolidation at both lung bases, as well as some reticular changes in the left lower lobe. CT of the chest image in lung windows showed central peribronchial interstitial thickening with some mild peribronchial nodularity evident.

Diagnosis: CIP.

Discussion: CIP refers to a diffuse inflammatory process of the pulmonary interlobular and perivascular/peribronchial interstitium. Entities that are included in the category of CIP include IPF, drug-related CIP, postinfectious etiologies, pneumoconiosis, and collagen vascular disease–related CIP. The offending agent in this case was never isolated, but pathologic features suggested that the CIP in this case was most likely postviral infection in etiology, and less likely a drug reaction.

The radiographic features are similar in each case, resembling that of IPF. An acute alveolitis may be seen initially, which may either resolve or progress to interstitial fibrosis. In the more chronic phase of fibrosis, HRCT findings include thickening of the peripheral interlobular septa seen as short interstitial lines, as well as longer, thicker parenchymal bands that generally extend out to the pleural surface.

CASE 54

History: A 34-year old white woman with a history of alveolar proteinosis and nocardia pulmonary abscess presented with a worsening cough productive of yellow sputum, pleuritic chest pain, fever, and nausea and vomiting. Alveolar proteinosis had been diagnosed on lung biopsy during a previous admission.

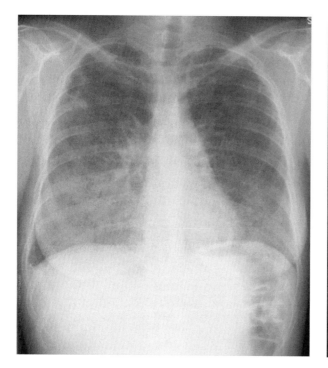

Figure 54A

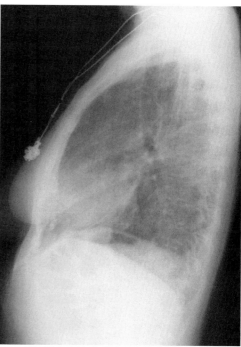

Figure 54B

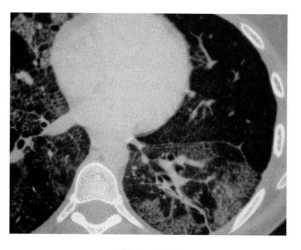

Figure 54C

Findings: PA and lateral chest radiographs show diffuse coarse reticular changes, with more focal consolidation at the right lung base. Cystic changes are also noted in the apices. HRCT of the chest showed bilateral patchy ground-glass changes and interstitial thickening. Cystic changes were also seen bilaterally. There was scarring and retraction in the area of the left lower lobe that previously contained the nocardia abscess. There was no focal consolidation, cavitation, or effusion.

Diagnosis: Pulmonary alveolar proteinosis.

Discussion: Pulmonary alveolar proteinosis is a rare lung disease that occurs in about 1 in 1 million people. It has a male:female preponderance of 3:1. Its peak incidence is in the third or fourth decade of life. Respiratory manifestations are insidious in onset, with dyspnea and cough presenting as the most common symptoms. In the majority of cases, the etiology is unknown. However, when a specific cause has been found, it is known as secondary pulmonary alveolar proteinosis. Secondary causes include immunodeficient states such as hematologic malignancies, and exposure to chemical or mineral dusts.

On plain films, there may be a geographic pattern of airspace consolidation, which is characteristic for this disease process. The consolidation is bilateral, patchy, and variable in distribution. There are reports of a perihilar distribution of disease in 50% of patients. In 20% of cases, the pattern is asymmetric, and occasionally isolated lobar involvement is noted. HRCT shows diffuse airspace consolidation, and thickened interlobular septa within the opacification, producing a crazy-paving pattern. Air bronchograms are not usually seen, even though there is significant alveolar consolidation. The crazy-paving pattern of disease is well demonstrated in case 31.

Patients with alveolar proteinosis are at risk for opportunistic infections such as nocardia, *Mycobacterium* species, fungal disease, or *Pneumocystis carinii* due to impaired macrophage function. Infections can cause superimposed radiographic changes, including cavities, nodules, and interstitial thickening. CT can assist in finding local areas of consolidation or abscess formation that may confirm the clinical suspicion of superimposed infection.

Treatment consists of whole lung lavage with an overall excellent but variable prognosis. Some patients have spontaneous resolution.

CASE 55

History: A 65-year-old woman with a history of chronic atrial fibrillation had been treated medically for the preceding 3 years, and developed increasing dyspnea during an inpatient evaluation for diarrhea.

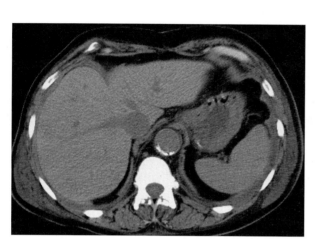

Figure 55A

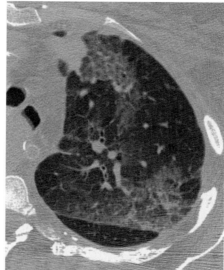

Figure 55B

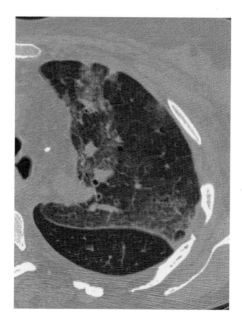

Figure 55C

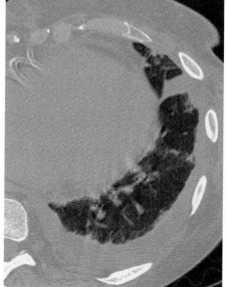

Figure 55D

Findings: There were patchy areas of airspace disease in the left upper, right upper, right middle, and right lower lung regions. There was mild bronchiectasis in the right upper, middle, and lower lung regions. Mediastinum showed no masses or adenopathy. Bilateral pleural effusions with associated atelectasis of the lung bases were noted. An incidental note was made of a right aortic arch with an aberrant left subclavian artery origin at the proximal right descending aorta. CT of the upper abdomen without contrast (A) demonstrated an abnormally high attenuation of the liver, consistent with hepatic involvement from amiodarone toxicity. The admission chest radiograph was free of infiltrates and effusions.

Differential Diagnosis: Hospital-acquired pneumonia is the most common cause of pulmonary infiltrates. Other possibilities include BOOP, aspiration pneumonia, hypersensitivity pneumonitis, eosinophilic pneumonia, and cardiogenic pulmonary edema.

Diagnosis: Amiodarone pulmonary toxicity.

Discussion: Amiodarone is an iodinated benzofuran compound that is being widely used for the treatment of cardiac arrhythmias such as atrial fibrillation, supraventricular tachycardia, and ventricular arrhythmias. The incidence of pulmonary toxicity varies from 0 to 60%, with an estimated mortality rate of 5% to 10%.

There are two types of presentation of amiodarone pulmonary toxicity. The first is more common, with an insidious onset of nonproductive cough, dyspnea, weight loss, and associated parenchymal infiltrates, predominantly in a diffuse interstitial pattern. The chest radiograph almost always correlates with the patient's symptoms. This type of presentation rarely begins before 2 months on therapy. The second type of presentation occurs in about one third of patients, is difficult to diagnose, and is associated with acute onset onset of symptoms. The chest radiograph shows an alveolar pattern with a patchy distribution and peripheral involvement. Patients with acute onset of symptoms develop fevers, dyspnea, and nonproductive cough and chest pain. Because these symptoms develop acutely, other etiologies such as infectious pneumonia, pulmonary embolism, and congestive heart failure are considered instead of amiodarone pulmonary toxicity.

The chest radiograph findings, although nonspecific in nature, play a key role in the initial suggestion of amiodarone pulmonary toxicity. However, one must be aware of multiple manifestations of this drug-induced lung disease. The predominant abnormalities seen on CT are diffuse patchy alveolar infiltrates with a peripheral distribution and rare association with pleural effusions. CT offers a unique opportunity to detect amiodarone toxicity, because amiodarone contains iodine that then accumulates in the lung tissue, giving it a hyperdense appearance. Thus, if the parenchymal density is increased on a noncontrasted scan, then it is suggestive of amiodarone pulmonary toxicity in the appropriate clinical setting. Further diagnostic intervention is warranted to exclude other causes of the parenchymal abnormalities.

The primary treatment of amiodarone pulmonary toxicity is discontinuation of the drug. The symptoms begin to resolve quickly in patients who developed acute pulmonary toxicity, whereas the resolution of symptoms is much slower in those who developed insidious onset of symptoms. Steroids have been used when patients have severe symptoms such as dyspnea and hypoxemia. Other possibilities include lowering the drug dose if the patient has life-threatening arrhythmias and the only treatment option is limited to amiodarone.

CASE 56

History: A 35-year-old woman with a history of end-stage renal disease from glomerulonephritis presented for a presurgery renal transplantation workup.

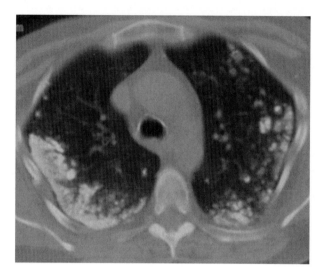

Figure 56

Findings: A single axial view from a noncontrast CT of the chest showed extensive high-density material throughout the lungs from diffuse calcification. The calcification was evident more in the peripheral region of the lungs than centrally. Although some of the areas of calcification had a nodular appearance, as in the left upper lobe, other areas, such as the right upper lobe, showed a more confluent area of involvement.

Differential Diagnosis: Differential diagnostic considerations for diffuse lung calcifications include hyperparathyroidism, silicosis, stannosis, pulmonary microlithiasis, pulmonary ossification from long-term mitral valve disease, granulomatous disease from TB or fungal infection, postinflammatory findings from prior varicella infection, and diffuse metastatic disease from osterosarcoma or chondrosarcoma.

Diagnosis: Diffuse calcinosis from secondary hyperparathyroidism from end stage renal disease.

Discussion: Diffuse calcifications can occur in the lung, as well as other organs, from primary or secondary hyperparathyroidism. Although this finding is not commonly seen, it is probably most commonly encountered with secondary hyperparathyroidism related to chronic renal failure (as in this patient), which is one of the more common causes of hyperparathyroidism. The calcifications seen with secondary hyperparathyroidism may have a coalescent appearance (as in the right upper lobe of this patient) or a more patchy distribution (as in the left upper lobe of this patient).

CASE 57

History: A 47-year-old male smoker with a history of fevers, weight loss, fatigue, and dyspnea had multiple small upper lobe cavities evident on CT performed at an outside facility.

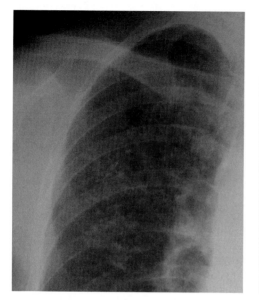

Figure 57A

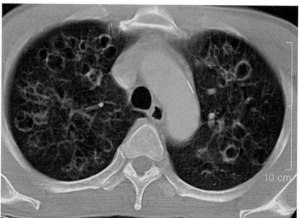

Figure 57B

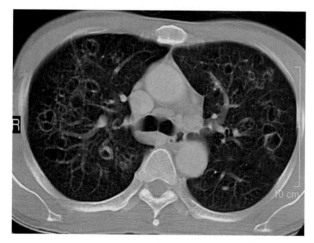

Figure 57C

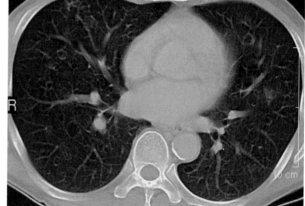

Figure 57D

Findings: A cone-down view of the right upper lung field showed diffuse cystic changes of the right upper lobe with nodularity. CT of the chest in lung windows showed extensive upper lobe cystic changes with minimal involvement of the lower lobes. The cysts were of variable size and wall thickness.

Differential Diagnosis: Multiple cavities in the upper lobes may represent emphysema, Wegener granulomatosis, EG, tuberculous infection, or bronchiectatic changes.

Diagnosis: EG.

Discussion: EG is also known as histiocytosis X and Langerhans cell granulomatosis. This is a multisystem disease characterized by granulomatous infiltration of the lungs, bone, skin, lymph nodes, brain, and endocrine glands. Pulmonary EG is part of a spectrum of histiocytoses that includes Letterer-Siwe disease and Hand-Schuller-Christian disease. These latter two entities are more generalized forms of histiocytic infiltration and are primarily seen in children.

Eosinophilic granuloma is an uncommon interstitial lung disorder that is strongly associated with smoking and is considered a smoking-related lung disease. It is an uncommon condition, with a slight male predominance, that occurs in young or middle-aged adults presenting with nonspecific symptoms of cough and dyspnea. Chest radiographic findings predominantly involve the upper lung zones, with an indistinct nodular pattern evident early in the disease process. As the disease progresses, a reticular interstitial pattern occurs, eventually developing into end-stage honeycomb lung. Honeycombing with end-stage fibrosis is seen only in a minority of patients with long-standing disease.

High-resolution CT is the preferred imaging modality for demonstrating the extent of pulmonary involvement. The characteristic features are nodules and thin-walled cysts. The nodules are usually less than 5 mm in diameter, with some noted in a centrilobular or peribronchiolar distribution. The cysts have an easily discernible wall of variable thickness (usually a few millimeters thick), and are usually interspersed within areas of normal appearing lung. The cysts are predominantly round but may have bizarre shapes from coalescence of several cysts, and they may be less than 1 cm to 2 cm in diameter. In almost all cases, the lung bases and the costophrenic angles are spared.

CASE 58

History: This patient was a 21-year-old smoker with recurrent pneumothoraces.

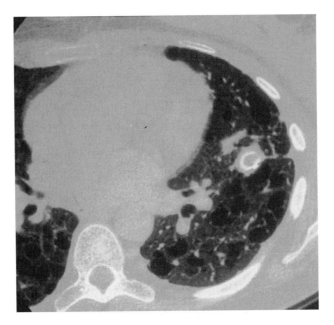

Figure 58A

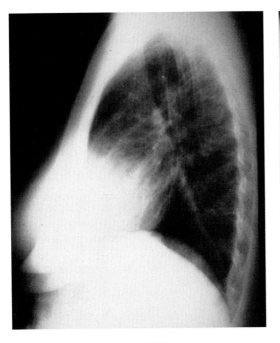

Figure 58B

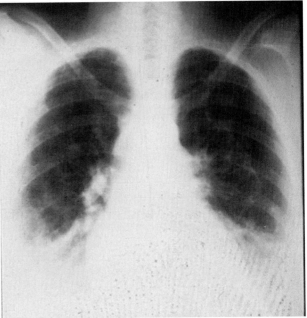

Figure 58C

Findings: PA and lateral chest radiographs and HRCT showed bilateral bullous changes involving the upper lung zones to a much greater extent than the left lower lung zones. The bullous changes varied in size from microscopic to larger cysts measuring approximately 2.5 to 3 cm in diameter. A left-sided chest tube had been placed and traversed the major fissure. No residual pneumothorax was identified. No pleural effusions or mediastinal lymphadenopathy were noted.

Differential Diagnosis: Cystic changes in a young woman with recurrent pneumothoraces is suggestive of apical blebs, emphysema such as α_1-antitrypsin deficiency, and LAM.

Diagnosis: Pulmonary histiocytosis X or EG.

Discussion: Spontaneous pneumothorax has been reported in 4% to 25% of patients with EG and may be the initial manifestation of this disease. A minority of patients have symptoms related to extrapulmonary involvement, such as pituitary or bony disease. Up to 25% of patients can be asymptomatic, but a majority of patients have a nonproductive cough.

During the early phase of the disease, primarily nodules are noted in the upper lobes. These nodules range from 3 to 10 mm in diameter and progress to thick- or thin-walled cysts. In patients who have only nodules, the differential diagnosis is broad and the findings often cannot be differentiated from miliary TB, sarcoidosis, silicosis, and metastatic carcinoma. Other abnormalities that can be noted are a diffuse fine reticular pattern, subpleural blebs, and increased lung volumes as opposed to decreased lung volumes seen with chronic interstitial lung diseases.

The prognosis is favorable when the disease is limited to the lungs, but patients have a poor outcome with multiorgan involvement. Complete or partial remission is seen in 13% to 55% of cases. The treatment of choice for EG is smoking cessation, with variable success noted with chemotherapeutic agents.

CASE 59

History: An 18-year-old woman who was a non-smoker presented with dyspnea and chest pain and was noted to have a pneumothorax on the initial chest radiograph.

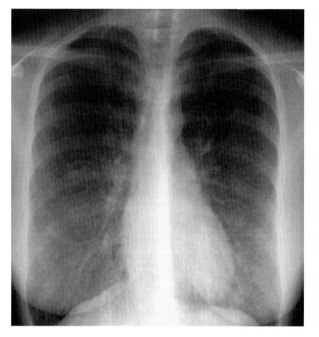

Figure 59A

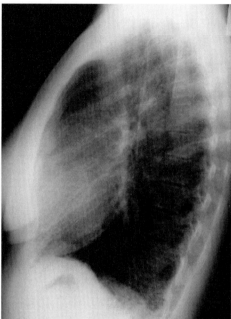

Figure 59B

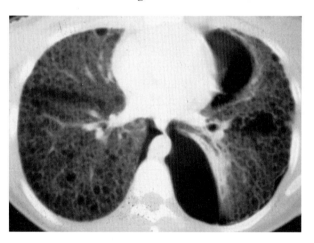

Figure 59C

Findings: PA and lateral chest radiographs showed increased lung volumes with diffuse cystic changes evident. A single image from CT of the chest better showed the diffuse cystic changes of the lung, with two areas of loculated pneumothorax on the left as well as a small pneumothorax on the right.

Differential Diagnosis: The differential diagnosis was limited in this patient, who presented with a pneumothorax with multiple cystic changes on HRCT. The differential diagnosis includes LAM, histiocytosis X, emphysema, bronchiectasis, and neurofibromatosis.

Diagnosis: LAM.

Discussion: LAM is a progressive diffuse interstitial lung disease of unknown etiology that occurs exclusively in women of childbearing age. It is characterized by atypical smooth muscle proliferation in the lung, pleura, and lymph nodes. The most common presentation is dyspnea on exertion and pneumothorax. Other common signs and symptoms include a nonproductive cough, hemoptysis, chylous pleural effusions, and chylous ascites.

The chest radiograph in LAM shows a generalized nonspecific, symmetric reticulonodular interstitial pattern, but with normal or increased lung volumes. Other disease processes that can mimic this pattern include hypersensitivity pneumonitis, histiocytosis X, sarcoidosis, and coexistent emphysema. The chest radiograph may vary according to disease severity, with some patients having normal radiographs early in the disease process.

The chest CT is nearly always abnormal at the time of diagnosis, but a better definition of lung parenchyma involvement can be ascertained from HRCT. CT may reveal diffuse cystic changes, which are thin walled and vary in diameter from 2 to 60 mm. The majority of cysts are distributed diffusely, and no lung zone is spared. These cysts are numerous and can be surrounded by relatively normal lung parenchyma. In some cases, a slight increase in linear interstitial markings, interlobular septal thickening, or patchy areas of ground-glass opacity are also seen.

The lung cysts in LAM are similar to those seen with histiocytosis X. However, several findings on the radiographs can differentiate the diseases: (a) small parenchymal nodules are characteristic of histiocytosis X, but are not common in LAM; (b) bizarre-shaped cysts are seen in histiocytosis X, and are rare in LAM; (c) LAM involves the lungs diffusely, whereas histiocytosis X occurs predominantly in the upper lobes. Other abnormalities seen on CT are LAM-associated lymphadenopathy, pneumothoraces, pleural effusions, alveolar hemorrhage, or lymphatic stasis.

Corticosteroids and cytotoxic agents have not been shown to be beneficial. There are anecdotal reports of response to hormonal manipulation, which include oophorectomy, progesterone, tamoxifen, antiestrogen agents, luteinizing hormone–releasing hormone agonists, and radioablation of the ovaries. Patients with end-stage lung disease have undergone lung transplantation, with actuarial survival rates of 69% at 1 year and 58% after 2 years.

CASE 60

History: A 60-year-old man with a several-month history of fevers, night sweats, and weight loss presented with a cough productive of yellow sputum.

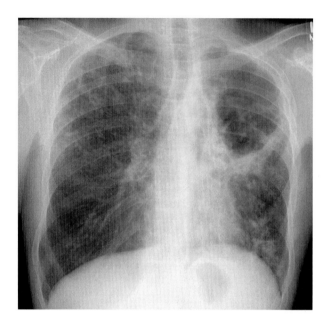

Figure 60

Findings: A single PA radiographic view of the chest demonstrated scarring in the left upper lobe with a large cavity. There was a diffuse reticular nodular pattern in the lungs, with more confluent airspace disease in the right upper lobe.

Diagnosis: Reactivation *Mycobacterium tuberculosis.*

Discussion: The hallmark of primary TB is the combination of a peripheral parenchymal opacity and hilar or regional lymph node enlargement. However, because most patients are asymptomatic, this stage may pass unnoticed. Subsequent radiographs may show calcified or noncalcified granulomas. The combination of parenchymal and lymph node granulomas constitutes the so-called *primary complex.*

In about 95% of patients, clinical illness is the result of reactivation of previous disease, years to decades after the primary infection. Typically, reactivation occurs in the apical and posterior segments of the upper lobes, but involvement of other segments and lobes does not exclude TB. The initial lesions are multiple small areas of consolidation and are often bilateral. If the infection progresses, the consolidations enlarge and frequently cavitate. Cavities are seen as rounded air spaces completely surrounded by pulmonary shadowing. In an untreated patient, a cavity is synonymous with disease activity. In untreated TB, the wall of the cavity is moderately thick. With treatment, the wall becomes paper thin but a persistent air-filled cystic space may remain. At some point, the cavities may be colonized by various fungi.

Reactivation TB also can take the form of lower or middle lobe bronchopneumonia. As with the primary form, it may spread to give widespread bronchopneumonia or miliary TB. Pleural effusions are frequent; they often leave permanent pleural thickening that may calcify. Hilar or mediastinal lymphadenopathy is uncommon in reactivation TB.

SUGGESTED READING

Abehsera M, Valeyre D, Grenier P, et al. Sarcoidosis with pulmonary fibrosis: CT patterns and correlation with pulmonary function. *AJR Am J Roentgenol* 2000;174:1751–1757.

Akira M, Inoue G, Yamamoto S, et al. Non-specific interstitial pneumonia: findings on sequential CT scans of nine patients. *Thorax* 2000; 55:854–859.

Akira M, Yamamoto S, Hara S, et al. Serial computed tomographic evaluation in desquamative interstitial pneumonia. *Thorax* 1997;52: 333–337.

Bartz RR, Stern EJ. Airways obstruction in patients with sarcoidosis: expiratory CT scan findings. *J Thorac Imaging* 2000;15:285–289.

Bicknell SG, Mason AC. Wegener's granulomatosis presenting as cryptogenic fibrosing alveolitis on CT. *Clin Radiol* 2000;55:890–891.

Damry N, Hottat N, Azzi N, et al. Unusual findings in two cases of Langerhans' cell histiocytosis. *Pediatr Radiol* 2000;30:196–199.

Flaherty KR, Martinez FJ. Diagnosing interstitial lung disease: a practical approach to a difficult problem. *Cleve Clin J Med* 2001;68:33–34, 37–38, 40–41, 45–49.

Hartman TE, Swensen SJ, Hansell DM, et al. Nonspecific interstitial pneumonia: variable appearance at high-resolution chest CT. *Radiology* 2000;217:701–705.

Kim EY, Lee KS, Chung MP, et al. Non-specific interstitial pneumonia with fibrosis: serial high-resolution CT findings with functional correlation. *AJR Am J Roentgenol* 1999;173:949–953.

Kim JS, Lee KS, Koh EM, et al. Thoracic involvement of systemic lupus erythematosus: clinical, pathologic, and radiologic findings. *J Comput Assist Tomogr* 2000;24:9–18.

Kim TS, Lee KS, Chung MP, et al. Nonspecific interstitial pneumonia with fibrosis: high-resolution CT and pathologic findings. *AJR Am J Roentgenol* 1998;171:1645–1650.

Lee JS, Gong G, Song KS, et al. Usual interstitial pneumonia: relationship between disease activity and the progression of honeycombing at thin-section computed tomography. *J Thorac Imaging* 1998;13:199–203.

Lee KS, Chung MP. Diagnostic accuracy of thin-section CT in idiopathic interstitial pneumonia. *Radiology* 2000;215:918–919.

Mampaey S, De Schepper A, Van Hedent E. Sarcoidosis. *JBR-BTR* 1999;82:117.

McLachlan MSF, Wallace DM, Seneriratne C. Pulmonary calcification in renal failure. Report of 3 cases. *Br J Radiol* 1968;41:99–106.

Michaelson JE, Aguayo SM, Roman J. Idiopathic pulmonary fibrosis: a practical approach for diagnosis and management. *Chest* 2000;118: 788–794.

Nishiyama O, Kondoh Y, Taniguchi H, et al. Serial high resolution CT findings in nonspecific interstitial pneumonia/fibrosis. *J Comput Assist Tomogr* 2000;24:41–6.

Patel RA, Sellami D, Gotway MB, et al. Hypersensitivity pneumonitis: patterns on high-resolution CT. *J Comput Assist Tomogr* 2000;24: 965–970.

Reynolds JH, Hansell DM. The interstitial pneumonias: understanding the acronyms. *Clin Radiol* 2000;55:249–260.

Seo JB, Im JG, Chung JW, et al. Pulmonary vasculitis: the spectrum of radiological findings. *Br J Radiol* 2000;73:1224–1231.

Shah PL, Hansell D, Lawson PR, et al. Pulmonary alveolar proteinosis: clinical aspects and current concepts on pathogenesis. *Thorax* 2000;55:67–77.

Sheehan RE, Wells AU, Milne DG, et al. Nitrofurantoin-induced lung disease: two cases demonstrating resolution of apparently irreversible CT abnormalities. *J Comput Assist Tomogr* 2000;24:259–261.

Sullivan EJ. Lymphangioleiomyomatosis: a review. *Chest* 1998;114:1689–1703.

Vos LD, Nollen AM, Gooszen HC, et al. Pulmonary histiocytosis X. *JBR-BTR* 1999;82:132.

Webb WR, Muller NL, Naidich DP. *High-resolution CT of the lung*. New York: Raven, 1992.

CHAPTER 4

CAVITARY LUNG LESIONS

MEGAN C. HODGE
PATRICIA J. MERGO

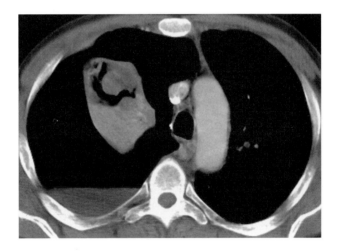

CASE 61

History: A 62-year-old white woman with a long history of steroid-dependent asthma, chronic obstructive pulmonary disease, bronchiectasis, and hypogammaglobulinemia secondary to combined variable immunodeficiency presented with a 2-week history of progressive worsening in shortness of breath and cough productive of yellow-green sputum. During the preceding year she had been diagnosed with *Nocardia* and *Aspergillus* pulmonary colonization and a right apical pneumothorax that required chest tube placement. Her initial workup included chest radiography, which showed a possible cavitary lesion in the right middle lobe. Chest CT also was performed.

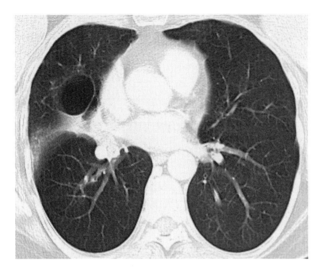
Figure 61A

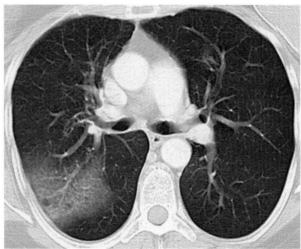
Figure 61B

Findings: Chest CT with contrast showed focal airspace disease involving the posterior right lower lobe, consistent with pneumonia. A 3.5-cm low-attenuation cystic structure with a thin wall also was seen within the right middle lobe.

Differential Diagnosis: *Staphylococcus* pneumonia, fungal or bacterial infection, cystic bronchiectasis, and bullae should be considered.

Diagnosis: *Pseudomonas* pneumonia (via sputum culture) with pneumatocele.

Discussion: Pneumatoceles are solitary or multiple cystic lesions secondary to obstructive overinflation associated with acute pneumonias. They also occur after lung trauma and hydrocarbon ingestion. They are most common in staphylococcal pneumonias in children, but are also associated with PCP in patients with AIDS. Pneumatoceles may occur and enlarge during the healing phase and eventually resolve within weeks or months without treatment.

CASE 62

History: A 19-year-old white man had been injured in a motor vehicle accident 3 weeks earlier. He had sustained splenic and liver lacerations and an L3 tranverse process fracture. CT of his abdomen and pelvis was performed to evaluate his liver and spleen.

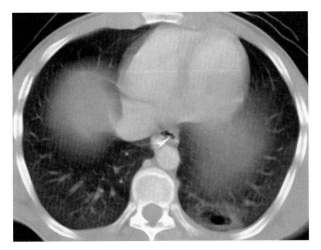

Figure 62A

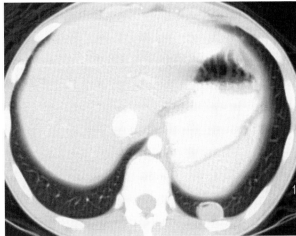

Figure 62B

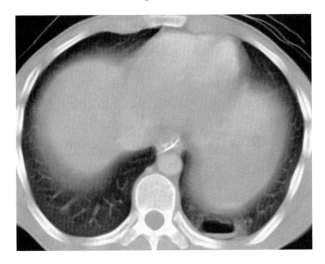

Figure 62C

Findings: CT of his abdomen and pelvis with contrast showed a small pocket of air in the left lung with an air-fluid level within the left lung base.

Differential Diagnosis: Posttraumatic pneumatocele and loculated hydropneumothorax should be considered.

Diagnosis: Posttraumatic pneumatocele.

Discussion: A posttraumatic pneumatocele occurs after blunt chest trauma. It is postulated that the shock wave causes shearing of a portion of the lung parenchyma with escape of air into the resultant fissure. This localized internal leak of air plus the retraction of lung caused by its inherent elasticity results in a localized rounded air space in the lung parenchyma. The pneumatocele may appear as an air-fluid level that later acquires a wall that, if bled into, will appear solid and indistinguishable from a hematoma.

Pneumatoceles can be solitary or multiple, uni- or multiocular, and measure 2 to 14 cm in diameter. They typically occur in a peripheral subpleural location immediately underlying the point of maximum injury but may be found elsewhere. Posttraumatic pneumatoceles usually disappear within 1 to 3 weeks, although some may persist a few weeks longer.

CASE 63

History: An 18-year-old white female college student who presented with left-sided pleuritic chest pain and shortness of breath. There was no history of trauma. Chest radiography showed a large left pneumothorax. Chest CT also was performed.

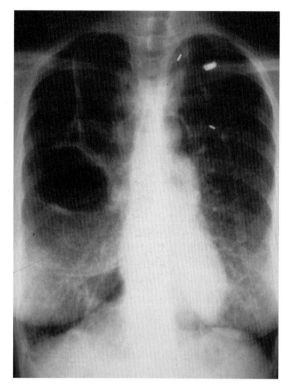

Figure 63A

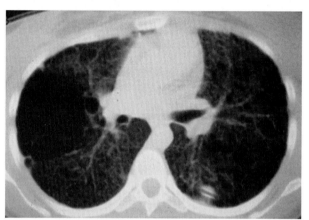

Figure 63B

Findings: A single PA view of the chest and CT of the chest without contrast showed marked, diffuse increased interstitial markings throughout both lungs. The lung fields demonstrated multiple small cystic lesions of varying size in a symmetric distribution bilaterally. Some of these cystic lesions have coalesced into larger lesions, especially in the lung bases in and around the cardiac silhouette. There were several large cystic spaces and multiple bullae bilaterally. There was also a large cystic lesion in the right mid-lung, as well as a large pneumothorax on the left lung.

Differential Diagnosis: LAM, sarcoidosis, and pulmonary tuberous sclerosis should be considered.

Diagnosis: Cystic changes of the lung and a spontaneous pneumothorax secondary to LAM.

Discussion: LAM is caused by a proliferation of smooth muscle within the lymphatics of the lung. It is a rare, nonfamilial disease found exclusively in women of childbearing age. In some instances, the thoracic duct is obliterated, resulting in chylothorax or chyloperitoneum. It results in well-defined uniformly thin-walled cystic spaces distributed diffusely throughout both lungs. With progression of the disease the cystic spaces enlarge and coalesce, reaching several centimeters in diameter and obtaining an undulating contour. Ultimately, honeycomb lung and chronic cor pulmonale are observed. Recurrent pneumothorax occurs in up to 80% of patients.

LAM should be distinguished from pulmonary tuberous sclerosis that has similar pulmonary pathology but is associated with low IQ, epilepsy, sclerotic bone lesions, adenoma sebaceum, and frequent renal angiomyolipoma. The radiographic findings in the chest, however, are identical.

The patient went on to experience repeated pneumothoraces and underwent pleurodesis and was eventually lost to follow-up while awaiting a lung transplant.

CASE 64

History: A 42-year-old black man with a history of coronary artery disease had sustained a myocardial infarction 9 years earlier. He had a 5 pack-year smoking history. He presented with a 1-week history of nausea and left arm pain and a 3-day history of fever and cough producing green sputum and a bad taste in his mouth. He had completed a 50-day jail sentence 1 month earlier. His initial workup showed a white blood cell count of 16,400 cells/mm^3. Chest radiography showed a cavitary infiltrate in the left lung. Chest CT also was performed.

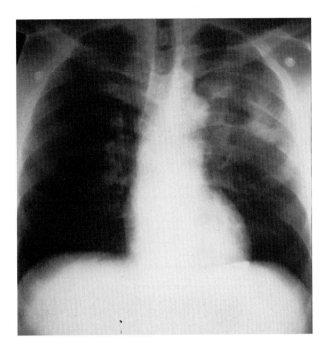

Figure 64

Findings: A PA view of the chest showed a 5-cm cavitary mass in the left upper lung. Its epicenter was at the superior portion of the interlobar fissure, possibly affecting both the upper and lower lobe. The mass had an air-fluid level and was surrounded by consolidated lung. The wall of the mass was thick and irregular, measuring approximately 1.5 cm. There was a small left pleural effusion and a few small mediastinal lymph nodes.

Differential Diagnosis: Lung abscess secondary to fungus or bacteria, TB, pneumonia, and bronchogenic carcinoma should be considered.

Diagnosis: Anaerobic lung abscess.

Discussion: A cavity is a gas-filled space within a zone of pulmonary consolidation, a mass, or a nodule. There may or may not be an accompanying fluid level. The features that have the most discriminative value in diagnosing the nature of masses that show cavitation are size, number, wall thickness, regularity and smoothness of outline, and position. Many of the causes of a single pulmonary nodule may result in cavitation, so the presence or absence of cavitation is not always of diagnostic value.

Lung abscesses usually have thick, nonuniform walls, with the inner and outer surfaces of the cavity being irregular. The tissue mass of the abscess has a wide range of attenuation values, including air, cavity fluid, parenchymal consolidation, and partially aerated lung. Viewing CT slices at lung windows is essential to study the abscess–lung interface and to distinguish trapped normal lung surrounded by pneumonia from a cavitating lung abscess. The interface between the main mass of the lesion and the adjacent lung is usually infected, creating a blurred, indistinct margin. The bronchi and the pulmonary vessels are not distorted or bowed by a lung abscess, but terminate abruptly at the wall, because the infection erodes into the surrounding lung.

CASE 65

History: A 54-year-old white woman had a 50 pack-year smoking history and a history of COPD with chronic, nonproductive cough. She presented with a 3-day history of "flu," with productive cough, fever, and malaise. She had a 1-day history of acute-onset right-sided back pain that radiated around to the right chest, worse with cough or deep inspiration. Her initial workup showed a white blood cell count of 15,200 cells/mm^3. Chest radiography showed a possible mass in the right lung. Chest CT also was performed.

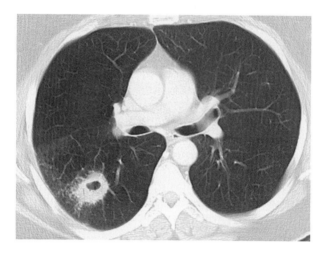

Figure 65A

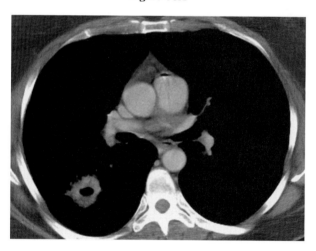

Figure 65B

Findings: Lung and soft tissue window images from CT of the chest with contrast showed a 3-cm thick-walled cavitary lesion within the superior segment of the right lower lobe. The lesion had ill-defined, shaggy, irregular borders with some surrounding airspace disease.

Differential Diagnosis: Bronchogenic carcinoma, lung abscess, TB, and Wegener's granulomatosis should be considered.

Diagnosis: Anaerobic lung abscess diagnosed via bronchoscopy biopsy.

Discussion: A lung abscess is a localized suppurative lesion of the lung parenchyma. It can occur with a variety of bacterial, fungal, and parasitic infections. The most frequent causes are as follows:

■ Aspiration of food/secretions (apical lower lobes or posterior upper lobes)
■ Infection beyond an obstructing lesion in the bronchus
■ Infected emboli, particularly in drug addicts
■ Necrotizing pneumonias

The hallmark of a lung abscess is necrosis or cavitation within an area of pneumonia or dense consolidation. Necrosis is commonly visible on contrast-enhanced CT as an area of low attenuation within opacified lung. Cavitation is present if air is visible within the lesion, and often CT is performed to confirm this diagnosis when the plain film is suggestive. Following cavitation, a thick wall with a shaggy inner lining is present in the acute stage and becomes smoother with time. An air-fluid level is common.

CASE 66

History: A 36-year-old white woman had a history of pulmonary hypertension secondary to underlying chronic lung disease. The patient initially presented 2 years earlier with dyspnea and chest pain. A ventilation-perfusion scan revealed multiple subsegmental perfusion defects bilaterally. An extensive workup to evaluate the patient for a hypercoaguable state was negative. Chest CT was performed to evaluate the patient for lung transplantation.

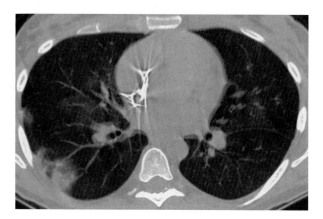

Figure 66A

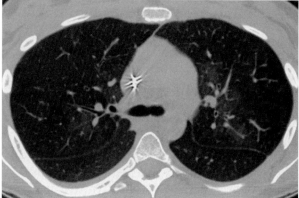

Figure 66B

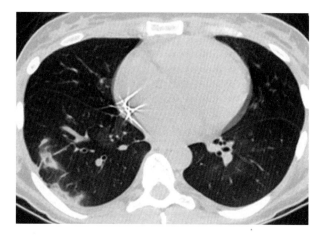

Figure 66C

Findings: Chest CT without contrast showed multiple patchy areas of parenchymal opacity that were more prominent in the periphery and adjacent to the pleura in the right lower lobe and in the left lower lobe posteriorly. Several of these areas were cavitary in nature. A patchy ground-glass appearance was noted more centrally in the perihilar region.

Differential Diagnosis: Chronic PEs, septic emboli, and pulmonary metastases should be considered.

Diagnosis: Chronic PEs.

Discussion: The clinical manifestations of pulmonary embolic disease are often nonspecific, ranging from no symptoms to presentation with sudden death. Typical signs and symptoms include dyspnea, chest pain, cough, hemoptysis, tachypnea, hypotension, tachycardia, fever, and a pleural friction rub. Most patients have an underlying cause, such as congestive heart failure, recent surgery or immobilization, or medications such as oral contraceptives.

About 10% to 30% of PEs cause infarction. Infarction occurs only when the combined bronchial and pulmonary arterial circulation is inadequate. Most infarcts occur in the lower lobes (corresponding to the regional distribution of pulmonary blood flow), and the majority are multiple. Pulmonary infarcts secondary to emboli are pleural based and wedge shaped, corresponding to the Hampton's hump seen on chest radiographs. Cavitation is less common than with septic emboli, but it does occur. Pleural effusion occurs in 25% to 50% of cases of PE. Effusions are more likely seen with infarction, and they tend to be small and unilateral.

Emboli usually resolve, and the vessel lumen is restored. When the emboli do not lyse, the presence of repeated, unresolved emboli may lead to chronic pulmonary hypertension.

This patient died 1$\frac{1}{2}$ years after CT was performed, secondary to pulmonary hypertension and right heart failure. She was on the list for a heart-lung transplant at the time of her death.

CASE 67

History: A 63-year-old white man with a history of severe peripheral vascular disease, DVT, and recurrent thromboembolic disease had undergone bilateral below-the-knee amputations. He also had a 50 pack-year smoking history. He presented with hemoptysis and right-sided pleuritic chest pain.

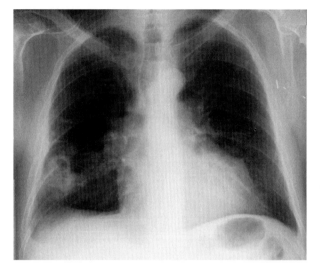

Figure 67A

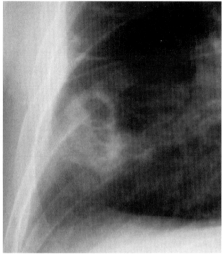

Figure 67B

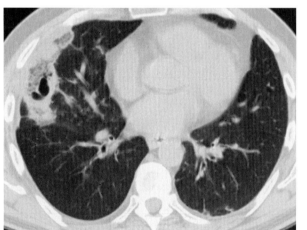

Figure 67C

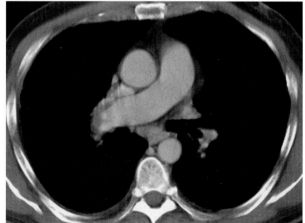

Figure 67D

Findings: PA and cone-down radiographic views of the chest showed a thick-walled right lower lobe cavitary lesion. CT with contrast showed at least three lesions within the right middle lobe. The largest lesion was a 4.5-cm thick-walled, cavitary lesion. The other two lesions were similar but were less than 1.0 cm in diameter. The large lesion was pleural based with associated pleural thickening. Mediastinal windows with contrast showed obliteration of the right pulmonary artery centrally from a large low-attenuation thrombus.

Differential Diagnosis: The patient's history of DVT and pulmonary embolism, combined with the symptoms of pleuritic chest pain and hemoptysis, put PE with infarction at the top of the differential diagnosis. The presence of cavitation brings up the possibility of septic emboli. Other etiologies that may give a similar appearance include pneumonia, bronchogenic carcinoma, TB, fungal infections, septic emboli, sarcoidosis, and Wegener's granulomatosis.

Diagnosis: Pulmonary infarction secondary to thromboembolic disease.

Discussion: Pulmonary infarction has a characteristic wedge-shaped configuration of consolidation abutting the pleura. The pleural-based density also may have convex bulging borders, and linear strands may extend from its apex toward the hilum. Scattered areas of lower density (necrosis) may be seen within the lesion. Infarcts may appear round, wedge-shaped, or truncated, and there is often a pulmonary artery branch leading to them. The appearance of cavitation within a pulmonary infarct may indicate a septic origin or secondary infection. After intravenous contrast administration, a peripheral rim–like area of contrast enhancement is often evident.

Other findings supporting the diagnosis of pulmonary thromboembolic disease include loss of lung volume with elevated ipsilateral diaphragm, oligemia, pleural effusions, and enlarged central pulmonary arteries with demonstration of the intravascular clot after contrast enhancement.

The evolution of an infarct is variable but reliable, indicating the nature of the consolidation. It may resolve within a few days or weeks depending on its size, age, and rate of lysis. An infarct usually regresses from its periphery toward its center. In the presence of tissue necrosis, the protracted resolution takes 3 to 5 weeks, and a permanent fibrotic scar may remain in the area.

CASE 68

History: A 49-year-old white man presented with acute onset of fever and mental status changes. Chest radiography showed a focal area of consolidation in the right mid-lung. Chest CT also was performed.

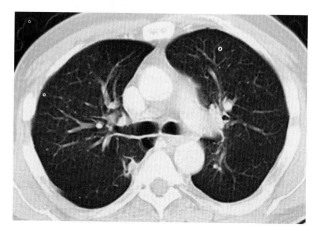

Figure 68A

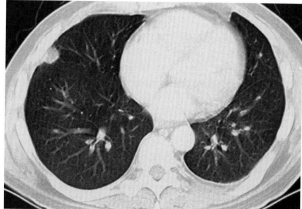

Figure 68B

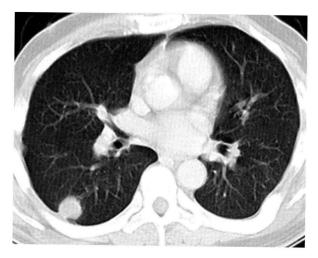

Figure 68C

Findings: Chest CT with contrast showed multiple pleural-based nodular densities in the right lung that measured 2 to 2.5 cm in diameter. A lesion on the medial aspect of the right lower lobe was cavitary in nature. There was also a small pleural effusion at the left lung base.

Differential Diagnosis: Septic emboli, pulmonary metastases, and Wegener's granulomatosis or other vasculitis should be considered.

Diagnosis: Septic emboli secondary to tricuspid endocarditis.

Discussion: Blood and urine cultures in this patient were positive for methicillin-resistant *Staphylococcus aureus*. An echocardiogram showed a 1-cm vegetation on the tricuspid valve.

Septic emboli are usually seen in patients under 40 years of age. They occur in association with episodes of bacteremia or septicemia. Bacterial endocarditis affecting the tricuspid valve is the most common source of septic emboli, but other predisposing factors include septic thrombophlebitis, indwelling catheters, hemodialysis shunts, osteomyelitis, intravenous drug abuse, and pharyngeal or pelvic infections. Organisms include *S. aureus,* gram-negative organisms, anaerobes, and streptococcus.

Pulmonary septic emboli usually present as multiple peripheral, ill-defined nodular opacities. They are almost always multiple with a lower lobe predominance. A wide variation in size may reflect recurrent showers of emboli, which occur in untreated patients. There may be a vessel leading to the lesion, air bronchograms, or associated pleural effusions. The appearance of pleural fluid may indicate development of an empyema. Cavitation is common, and usually relatively thin-walled, but thick walls with shaggy inner linings are not infrequent. An air-fluid level or a central density representing a piece of necrotic tissue (target sign) also may be seen. Finally, if endocarditis with valvular damage is the underlying cause, radiographic signs of congestive heart failure may be present.

CASE 69

History: A 56-year-old white man with severe ischemic cardiomyopathy was undergoing a cardiac transplant evaluation when he presented to the emergency room with development of grossly bloody sputum shortly after awakening. He also complained of dyspnea on exertion and orthopnea. He had a 2-day history of left-sided chest pain and denied any history of fever, chills, or night sweats.

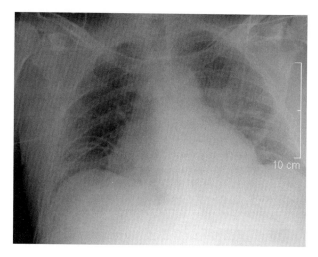

Figure 69A

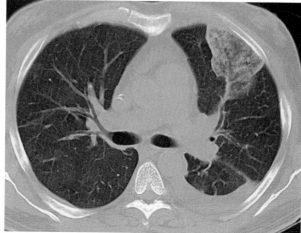

Figure 69B

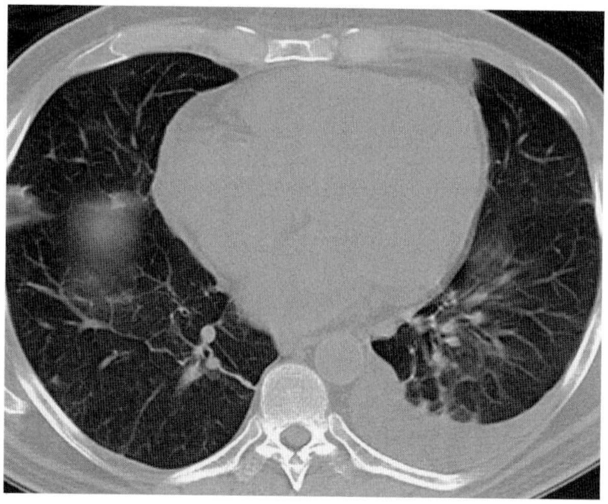

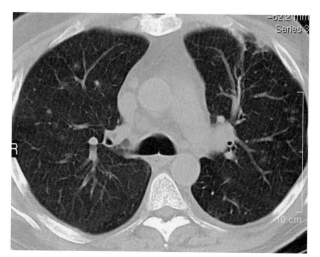

Figure 69C

Figure 69D

Findings: A frontal radiographic view of the chest showed an ill-defined parenchymal opacity in the left upper lobe with some suggestion of cavitation. CT of the chest demonstrated a well-defined, wedge-shaped area of airspace opacity containing acinar filling. There is an associated left effusion and a small cavitary lesion at the right lung base. Follow-up CT (C, D) showed near resolution of the findings in the left upper lobe over a 2-month interval with minimal parenchymal scar evident at the site of previous abnormality.

Diagnosis: Pulmonary infarction.

Discussion: In patients with suspected pulmonary embolism, the diagnosis of pulmonary infarction is suggested by the findings of pleuritic pain, hemoptysis, pleural rub, or infiltrate on chest radiography. Infarction is not an uncommon complication of pulmonary embolism, occurring in 10% to 33% of patients. Smaller emboli are more likely to cause infarction than massive emboli, and this may be related to the inferior ability of smaller pulmonary vessels to handle the reflex upregulation of collateral flow from the bronchial arteries. Underlying heart disease or chronic obstructive pulmonary disease is thought to predispose patients to infarction.

Airspace findings on plain films occur as a result of edema of the alveoli and hemorrhage into the alveolar space. The classic appearance on plain films is that of a cone-shaped infiltrate with a pleural base, as is depicted in this case. The apex points to the hilum and is usually rounded. The rounded medial margin is referred to as the Hampton hump and is a sign of infarction. Infiltrates are usually multifocal and predominantly in the lower lung fields. They are first seen 12 to 24 hours after the embolic episode. Air bronchograms are rarely visible on plain films, which may aid in differentiating the infiltrate from a pneumonia if this is not clinically obvious. Unlike hemorrhages, which clear within a week, the findings of infarction can take months to clear and often leave permanent linear scars. As it resolves, the infiltrate disappears from the periphery to the center ("melting away like an ice cube"). This again distinguishes it from pneumonia, which clears in a patchy fashion. An associated sign of pulmonary embolism is Westermark's sign of focal oligemia.

Cavitation in a pulmonary infarct is usually due to a septic embolus. When aseptic cavitation occurs, it is usually in an infarct greater than 4 cm in diameter. The cavity is first discernible about 2 weeks after the appearance of the infiltrate.

CASE 70

History: A 54-year-old man had a long history of asthma and emphysema and a 5-year history of *Mycobacterium avium-intracellulare* (MAI). He presented with recently increased shortness of breath and cough productive of blood-tinged sputum. He had had a 20 pack-year smoking history, but quit when diagnosed with MAI. Chest CT was performed to evaluate for bronchiectasis.

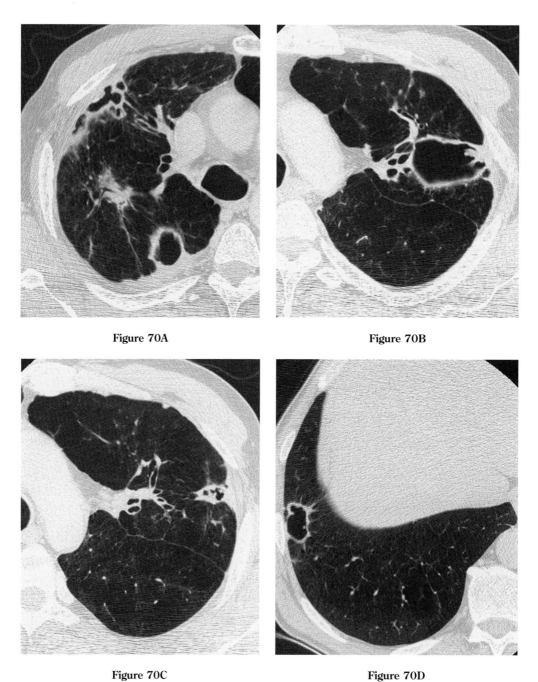

Figure 70A

Figure 70B

Figure 70C

Figure 70D

Findings: Chest CT with contrast showed chronic changes in both lungs with significant apical bullous and nodular changes and bronchiectasis in the upper lobes. There were bilateral apical cavitary changes and diffuse underlying emphysema. A peripheral and posterior right lower lobe cavity measured 2.5 cm in diameter, and a peripherally and posteriorly located left upper lobe cavity was two to three times larger. Reactive adenopathy was evident within the mediastinum, as was bilateral apical pleural thickening.

Differential Diagnosis: Bronchiectasis secondary to MAI, or other infectious etiologies, and cystic fibrosis should be considered.

Diagnosis: Bronchiectasis secondary to MAI in a patient with underlying emphysema.

Discussion: Generally, MAI occurs in men over 40 years of age with preexistent pulmonary and nonpulmonary diseases, including COPD, silicosis, and malignancy. It has become an important cause of pulmonary disease in patients with AIDS. It is not uncommon for the pulmonary disease to remain relatively stable without treatment and in the face of persistently positive sputum cultures.

Upper lobe cavitary disease is the usual radiographic presentation and it is thus indistinguishable from TB. However, bronchiectasis and cavitation (multiple) tends to be a more prominent feature of atypical mycobacterial disease than of *Mycobacterium tuberculosis*. These cavities predominantly involve the apical and posterior regions of the upper lobes and the posterior segments of the lower lobes. The wall of a cavity is usually of moderate thickness and has a generally smooth inner lining. The cavities are surrounded by either airspace consolidation or fibrotic changes with loss of volume and bronchiectasis. Pleural thickening is commonly associated, but a fluid level is rare. The fungus *Aspergillus fumigatus* may colonize old cavities to produce a mycetoma lying free within the cavity.

CASE 71

History: The patient was a 30-year-old black woman with a history of a cavitary *Mycobacterium tuberculosis* lesion 10 years earlier. Despite treatment, negative sputum cultures, and clinical stability, the cavitary lesion in the right upper lobe had been slowly enlarging. In addition, over the past year, the patient had noticed progressive dyspnea on exertion and mild hemoptysis.

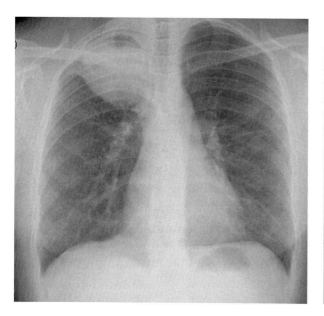

Figure 71A

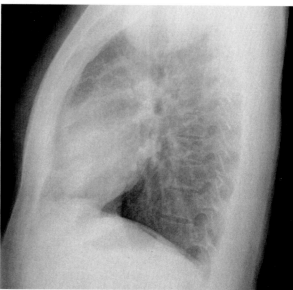

Figure 71B

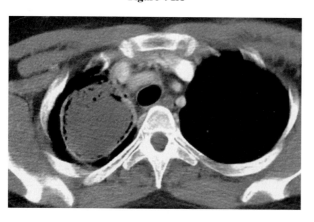

Figure 71C

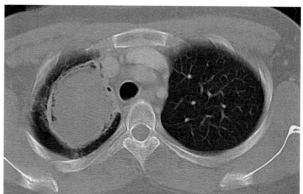

Figure 71D

Findings: PA and lateral chest radiographs showed a large right upper lobe cavitary lesion with a small air crescent near the apex of the lesion. CT with contrast in the soft tissue and lung windows showed a central cavitary mass in the right upper lobe, which extended up to the apex. It measured 6 cm in diameter. The mass had a cavitary nature with a relatively thin and uniform wall (4–5 mm). The mass was filled with soft tissue density material, except for a small crescent of air around the periphery of the lesion.

Differential Diagnosis: Mycetoma in an existing TB cavity, bronchogenic carcinoma, hematoma, and abscess should be considered.

Diagnosis: Aspergilloma.

Discussion: The infecting organism, usually *Aspergillus fumigatus,* is a dimorphic soil fungus found worldwide. The organism is a common finding in the sputum of normal individuals, with infection resulting from an altered host immune response or other predisposing factors. In general, four distinct manifestations of infections may be considered:

1. Mycetoma: Formation of a fungus ball occurs within a preexisting cavity, most commonly the result of TB, sarcoidosis, and bullous emphysema. This situation usually goes undetected unless the patient presents with hemoptysis. An opacity is seen within the dependent portion of a cavity, which shifts as the patient changes position. An air-crescent sign may be noted.
2. Invasive aspergillosis: This occurs in the immunosuppressed host. It has the appearance of a nodular opacity, with the formation of an air-crescent sign. Diffuse, rapidly progressive consolidation also may be seen. There may be a halo of ground-glass attenuation surrounding these nodules or infiltrates, secondary to focal lung infarction/necrosis.
3. Semiinvasive aspergillosis: This occurs in similarly immunocompromised individuals such as alcoholics, elderly debilitated patients, or patients with malignancy or radiation-damaged lungs. There is formation of a mycetoma within an area of cavitation after focal parenchymal infection and necrosis caused by the *Aspergillus* organism itself. Focal consolidation is seen initially, followed by cavitation and mycetoma formation.
4. Allergic bronchopulmonary aspergillosis: This occurs in chronic asthmatics in association with bronchial mucus plugging and dilatation. On chest radiography, it appears as tubular shadows caused by dilated, mucus-filled bronchi. Occasionally, a "cluster of grapes" appearance may be seen in cases of severe, cystic bronchial dilatation.

CASE 72

History: A 64-year-old black man with a history of hypertension presented with acute onset of tearing chest pain that radiated to his back. He was a truck driver who traveled extensively throughout the United States.

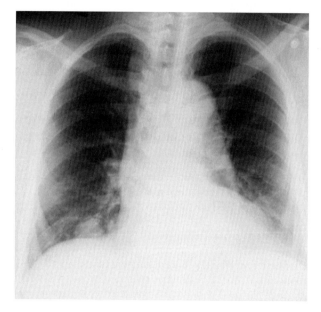

Figure 72A

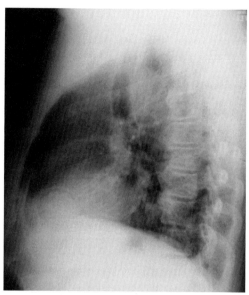

Figure 72B

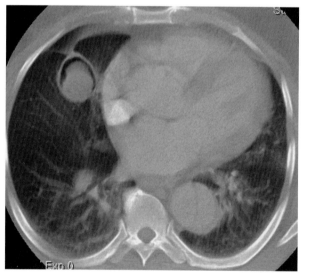

Figure 72C

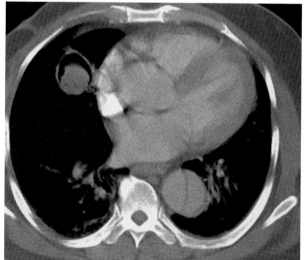

Figure 72D

Findings: PA and lateral radiographic views of the chest showed a widened mediastinum and a round, increased opacity in the right middle lobe surrounded by lucent lung. CT of the chest with contrast showed an aortic dissection that appeared to originate from the arch of the aorta and to extend inferiorly into both common iliac vessels (not the focus of this case). Within the lung parenchyma, there was a cavity within the right middle lobe and the presence of a soft tissue density mass in the dependent portion of this cavity. No mediastinal or hilar adenopathy was appreciated.

Differential Diagnosis: Fungus ball, bronchogenic carcinoma, and abscess should be considered.

Diagnosis: Fungus ball.

Discussion: In patients with a preexisting cyst or cavity, a mycetoma or fungus ball can form as a result of a saprophytic infection, usually by *Aspergillus.* On CT, a round or oval mass can be seen within the cavity, in a dependent location, and is typically mobile when the patient changes position. Air is seen between the mycetoma and the wall of the cavity (air-crescent sign). Thickening of the cavity wall is common. In patients with a developing mycetoma, the fungus ball can contain multiple air collections.

Most patients with mycetoma are over 40 years of age and are more likely to be men. The fungus ball may be asymptomatic and discovered incidentally (as in this case), but hemorrhage and hemoptysis occur in 50% to 80% of patients. This patient's chest pain and presentation was related to his acute aortic dissection.

CASE 73

History: The patient was a 45-year-old black man with a 4-year history of sarcoidosis and a 4-month history of intermittent hemoptysis.

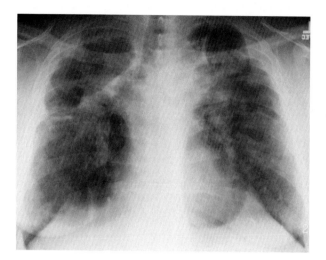

Figure 73A

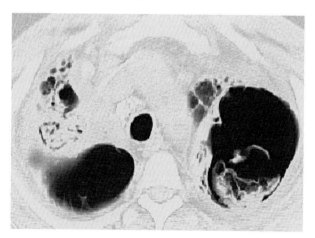

Figure 73B

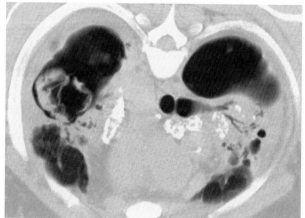

Figure 73C

Findings: A frontal radiographic view of the chest showed extensive fibrosis, upward hilar retraction, and calcified mediastinal lymph nodes. There was a cavitary lesion in the left upper lobe. CT of the chest without contrast showed a soft tissue mass or debris within a left upper lobe cystic cavity and some pleural thickening and consolidation at the right lung apex. Prominent paratracheal and bilateral hilar calcified lymphadenopathy and apical fibrocavitary changes were consistent with the patient's history of sarcoidosis. Supine (B) and prone (C) imaging of the chest demonstrated the dependent nature of the debris within the left upper lobe cavity. The debris is free moving, distinguishing it from a mass.

Differential Diagnosis: Considering the calcified lymph nodes and predominantly interstitial disease, sarcoidosis is the most likely etiology. The clinical picture makes interstitial pneumonia, silicosis, and tuberculosis less likely.

Diagnosis: Sarcoidosis with mycetoma.

Discussion: Sarcoidosis is diagnosed most frequently in black women 20 to 40 years of age. Approximately half of patients are asymptomatic at the time of diagnosis. It is staged radiographically as follows: 0, no demonstrable abnormality; 1, hilar and mediastinal adenopathy; 2, adenopathy associated with parenchymal disease; 3, parenchymal disease without adenopathy; 4, pulmonary fibrosis.

Parenchymal disease in sarcoidosis often predominantly involves the upper lobes. In patients with severe fibrosis, upper lobe cystic disease may develop. These cystic lesions usually develop on a background of diffuse reticulonodular pulmonary disease. An associated complication is the formation of a mycetoma in a parenchymal cavity, often found bilaterally. The mycetoma may cause severe pulmonary hemorrhage, a common and life-threatening complication.

The majority of patients with sarcoidosis of the chest have lymphadenopathy only. Bilateral, symmetrical hilar lymph node enlargement is a classic finding. Mediastinal lymph nodes, particularly the right paratracheal nodes, may be enlarged. Rarely, anterior and posterior mediastinal lymph nodes may be enlarged.

CASE 74

History: A 17-year-old black man with no significant past medical history was admitted for diabetic ketoacidosis secondary to new-onset diabetes mellitus. He was hypertensive and acidotic, and required intubation.

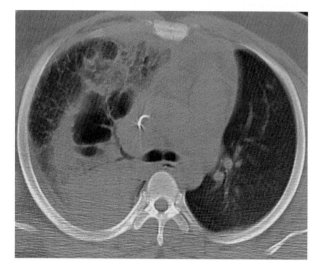

Figure 74A

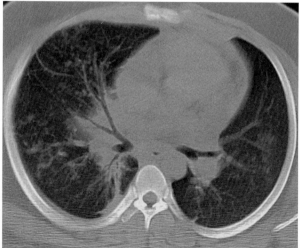

Figure 74B

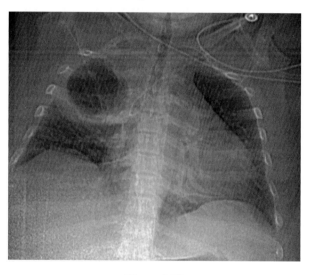

Figure 74C

Findings: A scout topographic image from a CT of the chest (*C*) showed a large cavitary lesion in the right upper lobe. Axial CT images (*A, B*) showed a necrotizing pneumonia involving the entire right upper lobe. Consolidation surrounded a central area of parenchymal destruction and cavity formation. There was also patchy airspace disease in the right middle and lower lobes and left lower lobe; a small amount of posterior pleural fluid was noted on the right.

Differential Diagnosis: Bacterial or fungal necrotizing pneumonia.

Diagnosis: Mucormycosis necrotizing pneumonia.

Discussion: Mucormycosis can cause a necrotizing pneumonia in immunocompromised patients. Mucormycosis has a 100% mortality rate in the absence of treatment and a very high mortality rate even with aggressive therapy. Approximately 75% of patients with mucormycosis have leukemia or lymphoma, or are immunocompromised from organ transplantation, and diabetes mellitus figures prominently among the remainder. Transplant patients are highly susceptible to pneumonia from mucormycosis. The most striking feature of the pathology of mucormycosis is fungal vascular invasion resulting in infarction. An inexorable centrifugal pattern of spread is common. This is characteristically seen with infection of the paranasal sinuses in diabetic patients, with frequent direct extension to involve the meninges and brain.

A single focus of disease in the lung is common, and this may manifest either as a pulmonary nodule or mass, or as an area of lobar consolidation. Cavitation is frequently seen and is probably related to vascular invasion by the phycomycetes with consequent infarction and necrosis. The cavity may contain a fungus ball. Foci of consolidation may be multiple and spread centrifugally with an ill-defined edge until the lobar boundaries are reached. Pleural effusions also can occur.

The patient underwent a right upper and middle lobe lobectomy due to the extensive necrosis but died postoperatively.

CASE 75

History: A 54-year-old black woman had a 6-month history of hypopharyngeal squamous cell carcinoma for which she had undergone radiation therapy. Chest radiography showed two masses in the right lung. Chest CT was performed to evaluate these masses.

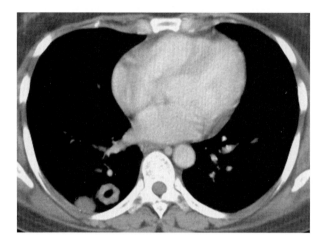

Figure 75A

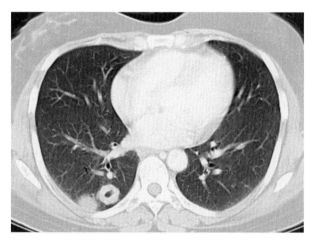

Figure 75B

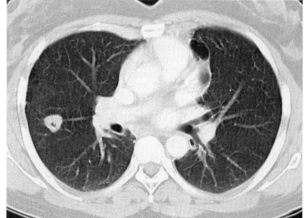

Figure 75C

Findings: Chest CT with contrast showed multiple thick-walled cavitary peripheral nodules in the right lung.

Differential Diagnosis: Metastatic neck cancer, granulomatous disease, lymphoma, Wegener's granulomatosis, bronchogenic carcinoma, and amyloidosis should be considered.

Diagnosis: Metastatic disease to the lung from a head and neck primary squamous cell carcinoma.

Discussion: Over 95% of multiple pulmonary nodules are the result of either metastases or tuberculous or fungal granulomas. The larger and more variable in size the nodules, the more likely they are to be neoplastic. On CT, the probability of multiple metastases is much lower and the chance of multiple granulomas is higher because much smaller nodules can be detected. Extensively calcified nodules are more likely to be benign, except in patients with osteosarcoma or chondrosarcoma, because metastases from these tumors frequently calcify.

Metastases to the lung are usually multiple, smooth, noncalcified, and peripheral. They vary in size and have to be almost a centimeter in diameter to be visible on chest radiography. CT scanning can demonstrate metastases as small as several millimeters in size. Pulmonary metastases may be seen to have a connection with a pulmonary artery branch, reflecting their hematogenous nature. However, this finding is also seen in Wegener's granulomatosis and bland or septic emboli. Associated hilar and mediastinal lymph node enlargement from metastases is less commonly seen compared to findings with primary bronchogenic carcinoma. Approximately 5% of metastases cavitate, most commonly from squamous cells of the head, neck, or cervix, and from sarcoma.

CASE 76

History: A 64-year-old white man with a 15 pack-year smoking history presented with a 3-week history of left upper and lower extremity numbness and a palpable left supraclavicular lymph node. He denied having respiratory symptoms. Chest radiography showed a large left upper lobe lung mass. Chest CT also was performed.

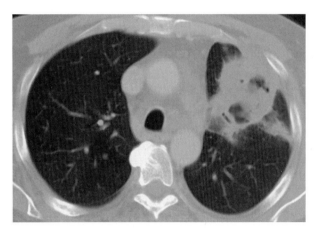

Figure 76A

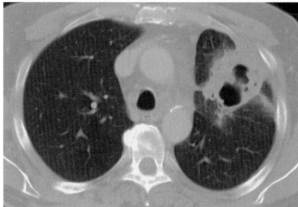

Figure 76B

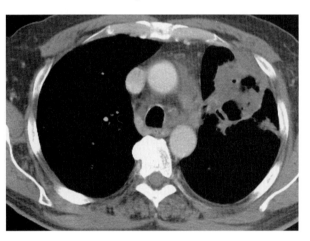

Figure 76C

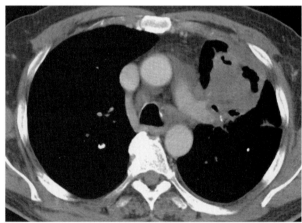

Figure 76D

Findings: Chest CT with contrast showed a left upper lobe lung mass with postobstructive consolidation and cavitation. The left pulmonary artery was partially encased by tumor, and there was mediastinal adenopathy.

Differential Diagnosis: Small cell lung carcinoma, non–small cell lung carcinoma, TB, and fungal disease should be considered.

Diagnosis: Non–small cell carcinoma (large cell type) with diagnosis obtained via supraclavicular lymph node biopsy.

Discussion: Approximately 25% of patients with bronchogenic carcinoma are asymptomatic at the time of diagnosis. Bone and brain metastases are often symptomatic at initial presentation, whereas liver, lymph node, and adrenal gland metastases are often asymptomatic.

Large cell carcinoma comprises 5% to 15 % of all cases of bronchogenic carcinoma. It is usually a large, peripheral, ill-defined mass. Large cell carcinoma is characterized by rapid growth, early lymphatic and hematogenous metastases (particularly to the mediastinum and brain), and rare cavitation (6%). When it cavitates, it is usually a thick-walled cavity with an irregular, nodular inner lining. Unfortunately, MRI of this patient's brain revealed multiple metastatic lesions, causing his neurologic symptoms.

CASE 77

History: A 54-year-old white man had a 66 pack-year smoking history and a 3-month history of hemoptysis. His initial evaluation included chest radiography with a right upper lobe cavitary lesion and diagnosis of MAI by sputum culture. He presented with a 3-day history of acute onset of shortness of breath, dyspnea on exertion, and right-sided chest pain. Chest CT also was performed.

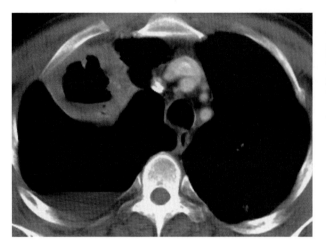

Figure 77A

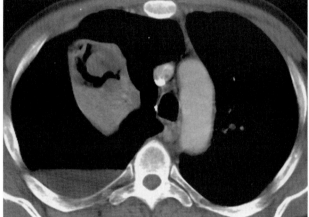

Figure 77B

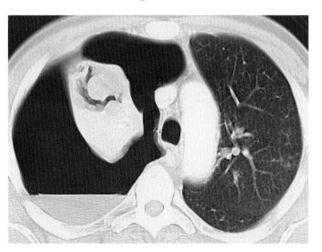

Figure 77C

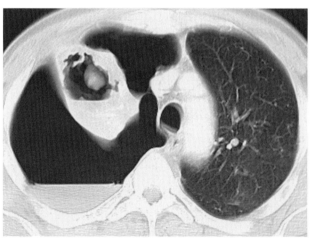

Figure 77D

Findings: CT of the chest with contrast showed a large right hydropneumothorax with a moderate amount of pleural fluid. A large right upper lobe cavitary mass was present. There was a mural nodule in the nondependent portion of this cavitary lesion. Several 1- to 2-cm pulmonary nodules were identified within the left lung. Multiple low-attenuation lymph nodes were also seen in the pretracheal region, consistent with the patient's history of MAI.

Differential Diagnosis: Primary bronchogenic carcinoma is the main consideration. MAI, and fungus ball could be considered, but not assumed.

Diagnosis: Squamous cell carcinoma diagnosed via transbronchial biopsy.

Discussion: Bronchogenic carcinomas often occur in the upper lobes, especially in the anterior segment. They occur in the right lung more frequently (3:2 ratio). Squamous cell carcinoma is the second most common subtype of bronchogenic carcinoma (25% to 30% of cases). The tumor usually arises centrally within a lobar or segmental bronchus. Central necrosis is common in large tumors; cavitation may be seen if communication has occurred between the central portion of the mass and the bronchial lumen (up to 30% of cases). Peripheral squamous carcinomas have the highest tendency for cavitation of all types of bronchogenic carcinoma. Distal airway obstruction occurs in one-third of cases, with segmental, lobar, or whole lung atelectasis. Pleural effusions are present in 10% of cases, and direct tumor extension into the chest wall, ribs, and vertebrae may be evident in advanced disease.

Compare this to a fungus ball, which lies free within the cavity. Air is seen between the mycetoma and the wall of the cavity (air-crescent sign), and the fungus ball moves around inside the cavity as the patient changes position. Therefore, on CT, a fungus ball should be seen at the dependent portion of the cavity, proven with supine and prone imaging, unlike this case.

CASE 78

History: A 42-year-old white man with end-stage metastatic lung adenocarcinoma presented with a 2-week history of hemoptysis and lower extremity edema. Doppler ultrasonography of his lower extremities showed bilateral deep venous thromboses. Chest radiography showed a left upper lobe mass consistent with prior studies and a new right lower lobe mass with cavitation. Helical chest CT also was performed.

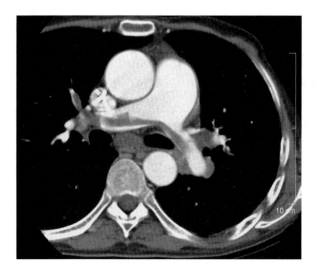

Figure 78A

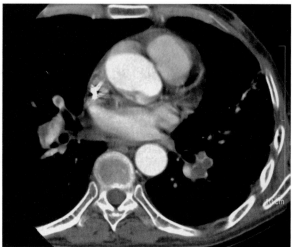

Figure 78B

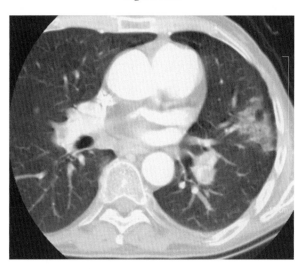

Figure 78C

Findings: Helical chest CT showed a saddle embolus in the main pulmonary artery that extended into the right upper lobe and left lower lobe pulmonary artery branches. There was an area of focal consolidation in the left lower lobe that was peripheral and wedge shaped in appearance. There was also a new focal, pleural, cavitary mass in the right lower lobe that is not shown here.

Differential Diagnosis: Primary bronchogenic carcinoma and pulmonary infarction secondary to PE should be considered.

Diagnosis: Adenocarcinoma of the lung with acute PE and left lower lobe infarction.

Discussion: Bronchogenic carcinoma appears as a peripheral or central mass, usually with irregular or spiculated borders. Distal airway obstruction presents as segmental, lobar, or lung atelectasis and obstructive pneumonitis in one-third of the cases. Pulmonary vessels may be occluded or contain tumor thrombi. Unilateral hilar adenopathy with or without mediastinal involvement is common and may be the only manifestation in 5% of cases. Adenocarcinoma is the most common type, occurring 35% of the time. It usually presents as a peripheral nodule or mass and cavitates only 2% of the time. This cavitation is usually thick walled with an irregular inner lining.

Spiral or multislice CT is now commonly used to diagnose acute PE. A filling defect visible within the pulmonary artery is diagnostic of PE. An acute PE is often outlined by the contrast agent, whereas a chronic PE is hard to distinguish because it is usually adherent to the vessel wall as it reendothelializes. The sensitivity and specificity of spiral CT in diagnosing acute PE in the main pulmonary artery branches approaches 100%, with an overall sensitivity of at least 90% when branches to the segmental level are included.

SUGGESTED READING

Baber CE, Hedlund LW, Oddson TA, et al. Differentiating empyemas and peripheral pulmonary abscesses: the value of computed tomography. *Radiology* 1980;135:755–758.

Bandoh S, Fujita J, Fukunaga Y, et al. Cavitary lung cancer with an aspergilloma-like shadow. *Lung Cancer* 1999;26:195–198.

Donnelly LF, Klosterman LA. Cavitary necrosis complicating pneumonia in children: sequential findings on chest radiography. *AJR Am J Roentgenol* 1998;171:253–256.

Gross BH, Glazer GM, Wimbish KJ. CT of solitary cavitary infiltrates. *Semin Roentgenol* 1984;19:236–242.

Jackson SA, Tung KT, Mead GM. Multiple cavitating pulmonary lesions in non-Hodgkin's lymphoma. *Clin Radiol* 1994;49:883–885.

Ichikawa Y, Fujimoto K, Shiraishi T, et al. Primary cavitary sarcoidosis: high-resolution CT findings. *AJR Am J Roentgenol* 1994;163:745.

Kazerooni EA, Bhalla M, Shepard JA, et al. Adenosquamous carcinoma of the lung: radiologic appearance. *AJR Am J Roentgenol* 1994;163: 301–306.

Maskell GF, Lockwood CM, Flower CD. Computed tomography of the lung in Wegener's granulomatosis. *Clin Radiol* 1993;48:377–380.

McAdams HP, Erasmus J, Winter JA. Radiologic manifestations of pulmonary tuberculosis. *Radiol Clin North Am* 1995;33:655–678.

Morgenthaler TI, Ryu JH, Utz JP. Cavitary pulmonary infarct in immunocompromised hosts. *Mayo Clin Proc* 1995;70:66–68.

Sider L, Davis T. Pulmonary aspergillosis: unusual radiographic appearance. *Radiology* 1987;162:657–659.

Staples CA, Kang EY, Wright JL, et al. Invasive pulmonary aspergillosis in AIDS: radiographic, CT, and pathologic findings. *Radiology* 1995; 196:409–414.

Tastepe AI, Ulasan NG, Liman ST, et al. Thoracic actinomycosis. *Eur J Cardiothorac Surg* 1998;14:578–583.

Yamashita K, Matsunobe S, Tsuda T, et al. Intratumoral necrosis of lung carcinoma: a potential diagnostic pitfall in incremental dynamic computed tomography analysis of solitary pulmonary nodules? *J Thorac Imaging* 1997;12:181–187.

LUNG NEOPLASMS AND OTHER MASSES

TAMMY EDWARDS KITCHENS
PATRICIA J. MERGO

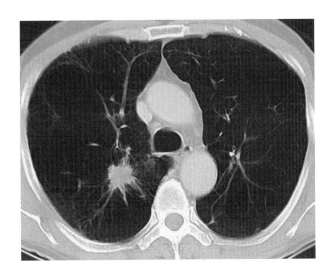

CASE 79

History: A 58-year-old male smoker with a history of smoking two to three packs of cigarettes per day for 40 years and a history of COPD. Chest radiography and subsequent CT of the chest was obtained as part of a workup for an exacerbation of his COPD.

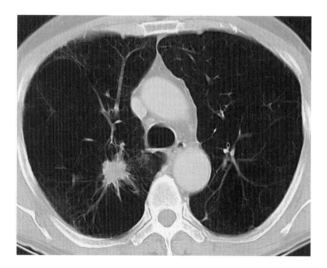

Figure 79

Findings: A single image from a CT examination of the chest showed diffuse emphysematous change throughout the lungs and a 2.5 cm spiculated right upper lobe mass with ill-defined margins and some surrounding ground-glass change.

Diagnosis: Squamous cell carcinoma of the lung.

Discussion: Lung cancer can arise from either alveolar or bronchial epithelium. There are four main subtypes of lung cancer: adenocarcinoma (35%), squamous cell carcinoma (30%), small cell carcinoma (20%–25%), and large cell carcinoma (10%–15%). These malignancies are often seen in cigarette smokers over the age of 40, with lung cancer now the leading cause of cancer death in both men and women. Although smoking is associated with greater than 85% of cases, other risk factors include previous radiation or radon exposure, remote and prolonged asbestos exposure, pulmonary fibrosis, and possibly viral illness. Radiologic findings highly suspicious for cancer include masses greater than 6 cm in diameter, solitary pulmonary nodules greater than 2 cm in diameter with spiculated irregular borders, unilateral hilar prominence, cavitary lesions with increased wall thickness (>1.5 cm), and persistent airspace disease.

Squamous cell carcinoma of the lung is the second most common form of lung cancer, accounting for approximately 25% to 30% of all lung cancers. This neoplasm has a strong association with smoking, may be associated with hypercalcemia and is locally invasive. The radiologic pattern most associated with squamous cell cancer is a large central mass arising within a lobar or segmental bronchus. This pattern is seen in about 60% to 75% of cases. Cavitation is common, especially in large tumors, secondary to central necrosis from keratinization. Peripheral squamous carcinomas have the highest tendency for cavitation of all types of bronchogenic carcinoma. Distal airway obstruction occurs in one third of cases, with segmental, lobar, or whole lung atelectasis.

CASE 80

History: A 53-year-old man with a history of smoking two pipes per day for 40 years had been treated for T4N0M0 stage IIIB squamous cell cancer of the left upper lobe 4 years earlier. He presented with new onset of fatigue, flu symptoms, and hoarseness.

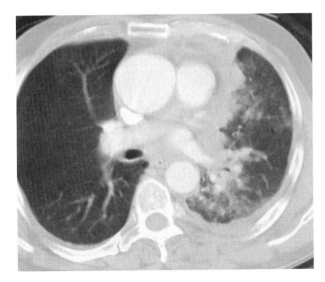
Figure 80A

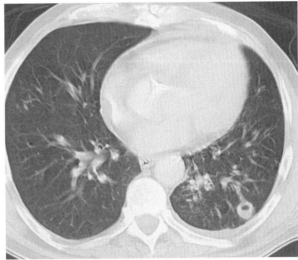
Figure 80B

Findings: Two images from contrast-enhanced CT of the chest showed extensive mediastinal adenopathy with extension into the central peribronchial interstitium on the left. Changes were evident from left post obstructive pneumonia, as well as a left lower lobe cavitary 1.6-cm mass.

Diagnosis: Undifferentiated small cell carcinoma of the lung.

Discussion: Small cell carcinoma of the lung is the third most common form of lung cancer, accounting for approximately 20% to 25% of all lung cancers. Metastases are common at the time of presentation. A poor prognosis is anticipated, with less than 50% survival at 12 to 18 months despite intensive chemotherapy. The radiologic pattern most associated with small cell cancer is a large central mass with extensive adenopathy. Ectopic hormone production with SIADH and Cushing syndrome is seen in approximately 15% of cases.

CASE 81

History: A 59-year-old female smoker of uncertain quantity and chronicity presented with striking sudden facial edema.

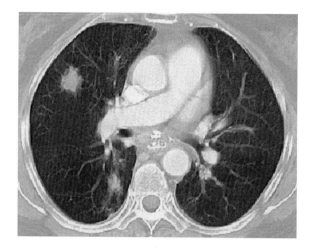

Figure 81A

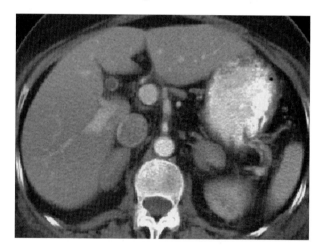

Figure 81B

Findings: Extensive mediastinal lymphadenopathy was present, with a large precarinal and subcarinal mass extending up to the right paratracheal region with compression of the superior vena cava (SVC) and left brachiocephalic vein. A focal pulmonary parenchymal mass was seen in the right upper lobe as well as a smaller nodule in the right lower lobe. CT of the upper abdomen showed bilateral adrenal masses that were not present on a previous CT of the abdomen.

Diagnosis: Undifferentiated small cell carcinoma of the lung.

Discussion: A pattern of disease frequently seen with small cell lung cancer is a large central mass with extensive adenopathy. The associated lymphadenopathy of the tumor can compress mediastinal structures such as the SVC, producing the so-called SVC syndrome. SVC syndrome is clinically manifested by severe dyspnea and marked edema of the face, neck, and sometimes the upper extremities. SVC syndrome also can be seen secondary to the massive lymphadenopathy from Hodgkin's lymphoma. This patient had SVC syndrome as a complication of her tumor, as well as bilateral adrenal metastases.

CASE 82

History: A 62-year-old man with a history of smoking two packs of cigarettes per day for 40 years presented with a new onset of a generalized tonic clonic seizure, frontal headache, and a large frontal lobe brain mass on CT.

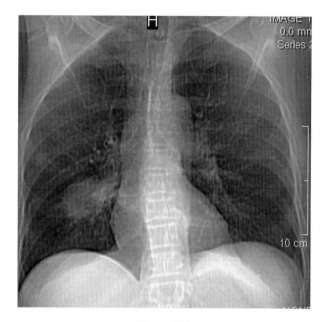

Figure 82A

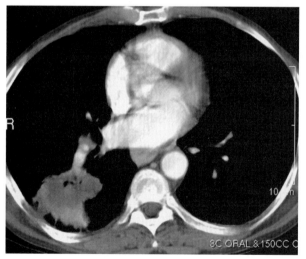

Figure 82B

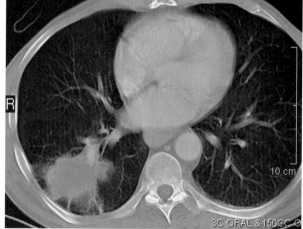

Figure 82C

Findings: A scout topographic image from a CT examination showed a 5-cm right lower lobe mass. Contrast-enhanced CT showed a right lower lobe mass with central necrosis, ill-defined margins, and surrounding ground-glass changes. Associated subcarinal adenopathy also was present.

Diagnosis: Adenocarcinoma of the lung.

Discussion: Adenocarcinoma of the lung is the most common form of lung cancer, accounting for approximately 35% of all lung cancers. It has a weaker association with smoking than other forms of lung cancer, and may be associated with prior lung injury or scar (scar carcinoma) and is more common in women than men. The radiologic pattern most associated with adenocarcinoma is a solitary pulmonary nodule, seen in about 55% of cases. Twelve percent of patients have a peripheral mass with associated lymphadenopathy. Also associated with adenocarcinoma is airspace disease with a radiographic appearance of ground-glass opacity. The upper lobes are commonly involved with this tumor, and cavitation is rare.

CASE 83

History: A 63-year-old man with a history of smoking one pack of cigarettes per day for 40 years and a history of asbestos exposure presented with cough and upper respiratory symptoms of 1 month's duration. Chest radiography revealed a new right pleural effusion, which thoracentesis showed to be of the bloody exudative type.

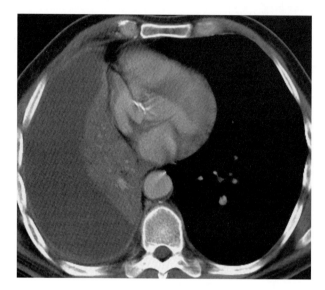

Figure 83A

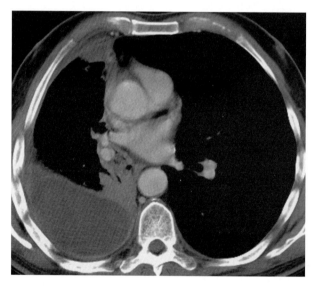

Figure 83B

Findings: CT of the chest with contrast showed a large right pleural effusion with some mild thickening of the pleura and a dense right lower lobe consolidation, with a more central right lower lobe mass seen in the region of the azygoesophageal recess.

Diagnosis: Moderately differentiated adenocarcinoma of the lung.

Discussion: Bloody exudative pleural effusion can be a secondary sign of malignancy. This case exemplifies the less common presentation of adenocarcinoma.

A known radiologic pattern of adenocarcinoma of the lung is a persistent pattern of airspace disease with air bronchograms. There may even be diffuse bilateral airspace opacities. All suspected "pneumonias" must be followed to resolution to ensure that the underlying process is indeed infectious and not malignant in nature.

CASE 84

History: A 59-year-old male nonsmoker with a history of adenocarcinoma of the lung 6 years earlier presented with recent onset of increased shortness of breath and an abnormality noted on a chest radiograph.

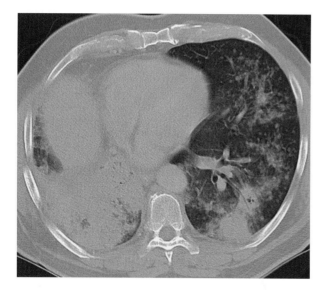

Figure 84A

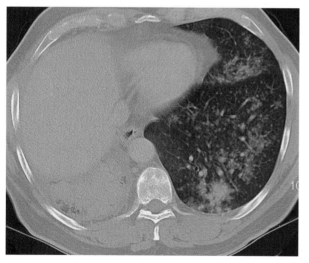

Figure 84B

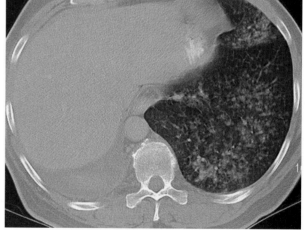

Figure 84C

Findings: CT of the chest showed extensive airspace disease in both lower lobes with multiple ill-defined parenchymal nodules in the left lung and dense consolidation of the right lower lobe with a right pleural effusion. In addition, there were innumerable tiny nodules throughout the left lung that extended along the peribronchial interstitium.

Diagnosis: Lymphangitic spread of well-differentiated adenocarcinoma of the lung.

Discussion: Lymphangitic spread of lung cancer or lymphangitic carcinomatosis results from tumor cells invading the lymphatics, which causes lymphatic vessel dilatation, surrounding interstitial edema, and a degree of thickening or fibrosis. The process often starts with hematogenous metastases to the lung.

   The radiologic pattern associated with lymphangitic spread of tumor is a nodular or smooth thickening of the interlobular septa and peribronchovascular interstitium that does not distort the pulmonary lobule. The interlobular septa are thickened out to the peripheral 1 cm of the lung, where their thickened appearance is often initially recognized. When this radiologic pattern is seen in a patient without a known primary malignancy, a transbronchial biopsy is often helpful in making the diagnosis. Lung cancer is a common cause of lymphangitic carcinomatosis and can present as a unilateral process. Extrapulmonary neoplasms that may also commonly result in lymphangitic carcinomatosis include those of the breast, stomach, pancreas, and cervix, typically with a more usual bilateral appearance.

CASE 85

History: A 48-year-old female nonsmoker had a history of recurrent bronchitis and pneumonia, fatigue, and occasional thick sputum.

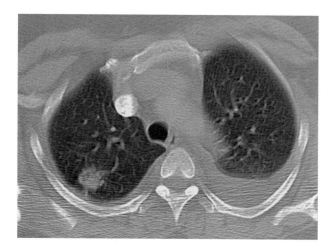

Figure 85A

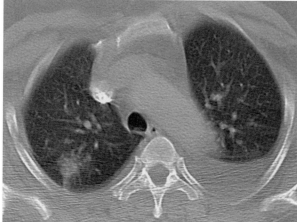

Figure 85B

Findings: CT of the chest with contrast showed a 2-cm nodule in the right upper lobe with shaggy, irregular margins and some surrounding ground-glass opacity. A large left effusion also was present.

Diagnosis: Bronchioloalveolar carcinoma.

Discussion: Bronchioloalveolar carcinoma is an uncommon type of adenocarcinoma thought to arise from type II pneumocytes and bronchiolar epithelial cells. It accounts for less than 5% of all primary lung cancers. It is not associated with cigarette smoking and does not have a gender predominance. It is most commonly seen in patients in the sixth and seventh decades of life and has a tendency to arise out of previously damaged or scarred lung tissue. The presenting complaint may be expectoration of large amounts of mucoid sputum produced by the tumor cells. This is termed *bronchorrhea*.

Bronchioloalveolar carcinoma most commonly presents as a solitary lobulated or spiculated nodule, often in a subpleural location, as in this case. Air bronchograms and bubble-like lucencies are often seen on CT, representing patent small bronchi. When it presents as a solitary nodule, it is more likely to be at stage I and is probably slow growing. Prognosis is thus relatively good. When bronchioloalveolar carcinoma presents as pulmonary consolidation, local spread is more extensive and metastasis is more common, resulting in a worse prognosis.

Bronchioloalveolar carcinoma also can present as multifocal areas of pulmonary consolidation. They may have any appearance, from ground-glass opacity to solid consolidation, with lobar to patchy, multifocal distribution. Pneumonia, aspiration, and pulmonary edema should be considered in the differential diagnosis. On CT, air bronchograms are common. As in the nodular form, a bubbly pattern of small, rounded collections of air due to patent bronchi and cystic spaces may be seen. Thickened septal lines, branching tubular densities, and mucoid impaction suggest lymphatic permeation. Pleural effusions and hilar and mediastinal lymphadenopathy are common.

CASE 86

History: A 51-year-old man with a history of smoking one pack of cigarettes per day for 20 years had lost 50 pounds. He had a 2-year history of a right renal mass, which had been decreasing in size over the first year of observation but had begun to grow again.

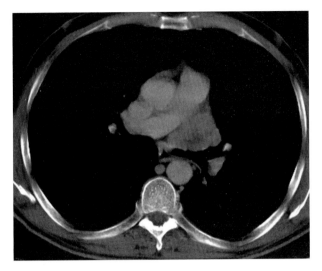

Figure 86A

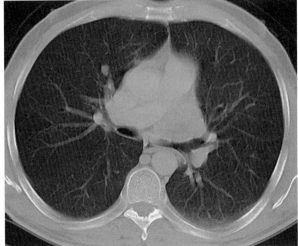

Figure 86B

Findings: CT of the chest with contrast showed a large left perihilar mass, just posterior to the left pulmonary artery. The mass narrowed the left upper lobe bronchus, as demonstrated on the lung parenchymal windows. Noncalcified lung nodules were observed in the right upper lobe (shown on the lung parenchymal windows) and right lower lobe. Bilateral adrenal masses also were present in this patient (not included in the images shown here).

Diagnosis: Large cell cytokeratin positive carcinoma of the lung.

Discussion: Large cell carcinoma of the lung is the fourth most common form of lung cancer, accounting for approximately 10% to 15% of all lung cancers. Metastasis is common at the time of presentation. A poor prognosis is anticipated. The radiologic pattern most associated with large cell cancer is a large peripheral mass, usually greater than 6 cm in diameter, that exhibits rapid growth. Central necrosis with cavitation may be seen.

CASE 87

History: A 55-year-old man with a history of smoking two packs of cigarettes per day for 40 years had mild shortness of breath and chronic nonproductive cough. Imaging of the chest was obtained in preparation for abdominal aortic aneurysm repair.

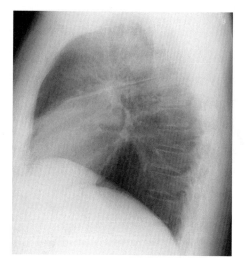

Figure 87A

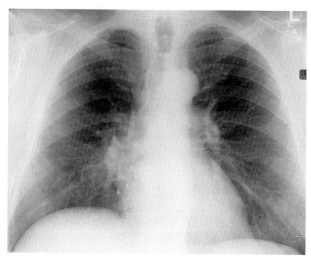

Figure 87B

Findings: PA and lateral views of the chest showed enlargement of the right hilum and infrahilar region. The patient subsequently underwent bronchoscopic evaluation.

Diagnosis: Carcinoid.

Discussion: Carcinoid lung tumors most often present as central endobronchial lesions with associated postobstructive pneumonia or atelectasis. Shortness of breath, wheezing, cough, and hemoptysis are common symptoms. Hemoptysis may be massive secondary to the vascular nature of these tumors.

Less than 20% of carcinoids are intraparenchymal lesions. These tumors are neuroendocrine in origin from amine precursor uptake and decarboxylation cells or Kulchitzky cells, and may secrete serotonin, vasoactive intestinal peptide, adrenocorticotropic hormone, or antidiuretic hormone, resulting in carcinoid syndrome. Carcinoid syndrome is seen in fewer than 3% of cases.

CASE 88

History: A 49-year-old female nonsmoker presented with increasing dry cough, wheezing, dyspnea on exertion, shortness of breath, fatigue, and pleuritic chest pain.

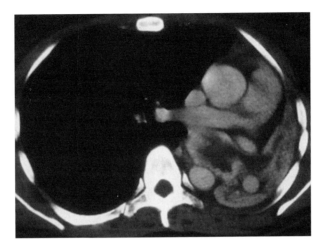

Figure 88

Findings: Contrast-enhanced CT of the chest demonstrated a 4-cm soft tissue mass with a hypodense center posterior to the left main bronchus. The mass caused total occlusion of the left main bronchus with atelectasis of the entire left lung, seen as an enhancing peripheral opacity in the left hemithorax.

Diagnosis: Spindle cell neoplasm consistent with carcinosarcoma of the lung.

Discussion: Carcinosarcoma of the lung is a less commonly encountered lesion, but one with an associated poor prognosis. Like large cell lung cancers, carcinosarcomas of the lung have a rapid doubling time of usually less than 1 month.

Interestingly, this patient elected to try an alternative form of treatment with high doses of the heavy metal germanium, ingested daily. The tumor mass shrunk subsequently, and follow-up CT examinations of the chest obtained for several years demonstrated no recurrence of the mass.

CASE 89

History: A 48-year-old female nonsmoker had a history of Hodgkin's disease treated with radiation therapy about 24 years earlier. She presented with new onset of chest pain, wheezing, and hemoptysis of 2 months' duration.

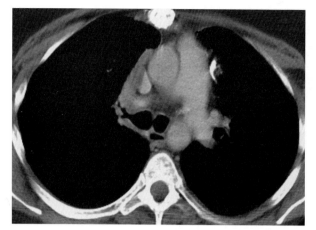

Figure 89A

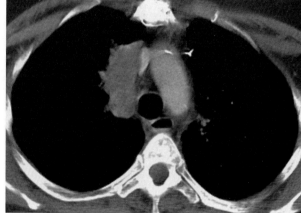

Figure 89B

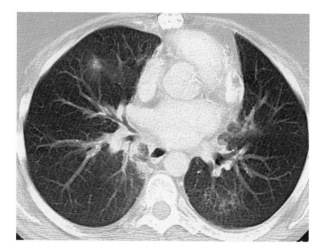

Figure 89C

Findings: Contrast-enhanced CT of the chest showed narrowing of the right upper lobe bronchus with some collapse of the right upper lobe. There was a small, ill-defined parenchymal nodule in the right upper lobe. Mediastinal windows showed a large right paratracheal mass. Although not included in the images shown, subcarinal adenopathy also was seen on the CT examination.

Diagnosis: Poorly differentiated non–small cell carcinoma of the lung, adenocarcinoma versus large cell.

Discussion: The diagnosis of non–small cell carcinoma is made as a diagnosis of exclusion if clear-cut pathologic criteria for subclassification as squamous cell, adenocarcinoma, or large cell carcinoma cannot be met. Therapy for non–small cell cancer versus small cell cancer differs drastically so differentiation between these two is critical for treatment.

The mainstay treatment for small cell carcinoma is chemotherapy, whereas the treatment for non–small cell carcinoma may include resection with curative intent, radiation, and possibly chemotherapy based on clinical staging. Although multiple pathologic criteria along with demographic data are used, disagreement among dedicated expert lung neoplasm pathologists for diagnosis of small cell versus non–small cell carcinoma may occur in up to 7% of cases, presenting a true treatment dilemma.

CASE 90

History: An 81-year-old female nonsmoker who was asymptomatic had a left lower lung abnormality noted on routine chest radiograph.

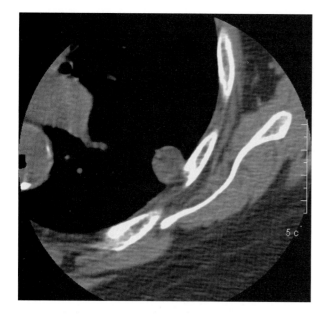

Figure 90A

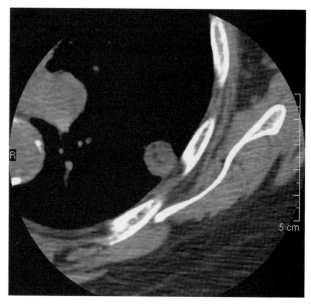

Figure 90B

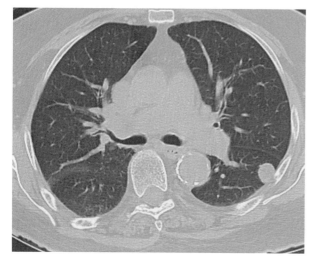

Figure 90C

Findings: Noncontrast CT of the chest showed a 1.2-cm noncalcified pulmonary parenchymal nodule in the superior aspect of the left lower lobe. Thin section imaging showed that the nodule had areas of low attenuation centrally within the nodule, consistent with fat density.

Diagnosis: Hamartoma.

Discussion: Hamartoma of the lung is most commonly seen as a solitary pulmonary nodule in the parenchyma (90% of cases) and presents as an endobronchial lesion in 10% of cases. This benign lesion is composed of fibrous connective tissue with varying amounts of fat, smooth muscle, seromucinous glands, and calcification or ossification. Multiple clumps of popcorn-like calcification within the lesion, which may be seen in approximately 30% of cases, supports the diagnosis.

Differential diagnosis of an endobronchial hamartoma includes a carcinoid tumor or other bronchogenic neoplasm. In the absence of visible fat within the lesion, this distinction is difficult to make by imaging alone, and may require surgical excision. Parenchymal lesions can be similarly difficult to diagnose if they do not contain visible amounts of fat. The differential diagnosis of a solitary parenchymal nodule should include granuloma, primary bronchogenic carcinoma, intraparenchymal lymph node, solitary metastasis to the lung, bronchial adenoma, lipoma, fibroma, round atelectasis, hydatid cyst, arteriovenous malformation, pulmonary infarction, amyloid nodule or other inflammatory granulomatous nodules (as seen with rheumatoid arthritis or Wegener's granulomatosis), lung cyst, and mucoid impaction.

CASE 91

History: A 65-year-old woman with a known cardiac history presented with sudden onset of crushing substernal chest pain. Chest radiography was performed as part of her evaluation, leading to further evaluation with CT of the chest.

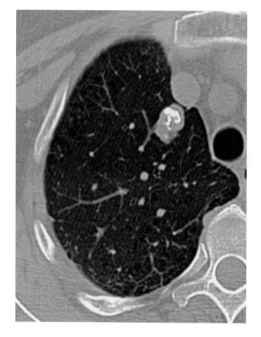

Figure 91A

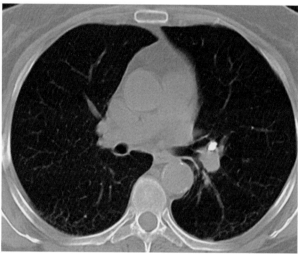

Figure 91B

Findings: High-resolution CT of the right upper lobe showed a small pulmonary parenchymal nodule with central stippled calcification. In addition, a calcified lymph node was observed in the left hilum.

Diagnosis: Granuloma.

Discussion: The differential diagnosis for a solitary pulmonary nodule was given in the previous case. Specific characteristics that may aid in defining a nodule as likely to be benign or malignant include the presence and pattern of calcification noted within a lesion, the rate of growth of a lesion, and, in the case of an arteriovenous malformation, the identification of a feeding and a draining vessel to the lesion.

Types of calcification that likely signify benign lesions include concentric or laminated calcification, which is specific for granulomatous infection from tuberculous or fungal infection, popcorn calcification, and diffuse or a uniformly dense appearance of a nodule from diffuse calcification. Popcorn calcifications are indicative of cartilaginous calcifications in lesions such as a hamartomas.

Punctate calcifications are less easy to classify and may be seen with either benign or malignant lesions, usually granulomas, hamartomas, amyloidomas, or metastases from either an osteosarcoma or chondrosarcoma. Primary bronchogenic carcinoma does not usually exhibit punctate type calcifications unless a carcinoma grows to engulf an adjacent granuloma.

Overall, CT, often with thin section imaging, is the best way to further characterize a pulmonary parenchymal nodule seen on plain film radiography. Noncontrast CT allows characterization and identification of calcifications within the nodule. Other features of a nodule also can aid in characterization as well. Recent work by Swenson et al. has shown that enhancement of a lesion can aid in predicting the likelihood of benign or malignant disease, with malignant lesions more likely to show enhancement following administration of intravenous contrast material. The shape of a lesion also can be used as somewhat of a predictor of malignancy or benign disease. Irregular margins, a lobulated or notched appearance, and the presence of fine spiculations emanating from a lesion giving it a corona radiata appearance are all findings that are more likely indicative of a bronchogenic carcinoma than a benign nodule.

CASE 92

History: A 34-year-woman with a history of smoking 30 pack-years of cigarettes had been on long-term immunosuppressive therapy with methotrexate and prednisone for an underlying chronic illness. She was previously noted to have a small nodule on chest radiography that had enlarged by 6-month follow-up CT examination. She also reported a 20-pound weight loss over the preceding year.

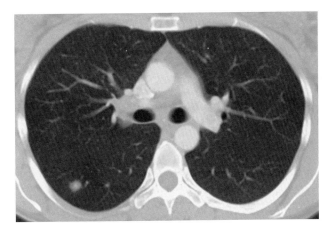

Figure 92

Findings: A single image from a CT examination of the chest showed a 7-mm nodule in the right lower lobe with some central calcification, but ill-defined margins with some mild spiculation. Because the nodule had increased over a 6-month period, thorascopic wedge resection was performed.

Diagnosis: Rheumatoid nodule.

Discussion: Surgical pathology revealed a necrotizing granuloma with changes consistent with a rheumatoid nodule. Stains for fungi and acid-fast organisms were negative. No malignancy was identified. The patient's chronic underlying disease was rheumatoid arthritis that she had had for 6 years.

Extraarticular manifestations of rheumatoid are more commonly seen in seropositive individuals. Pulmonary manifestations most commonly include pleural abnormalities, with a unilateral pleural effusion being one radiographic manifestation. Other pulmonary manifestations include diffuse interstitial fibrosis, rheumatoid pneumoconiosis or Caplan's syndrome, pulmonary arteritis, obliterative bronchiolitis, and rarely necrobiotic nodules.

The rheumatoid nodules are necrotizing granulomatous nodules that can reach a size of several centimeters and may be multiple. They are often seen in the periphery of the lung and can have central cavitation.

CASE 93

History: A 61-year-old man with known previous asbestosis exposure and a history of smoking 15 pack-years had undergone routine chest radiography as part of a workup for hypertension, as well as subsequent CT of the chest, with multiple follow-up examinations.

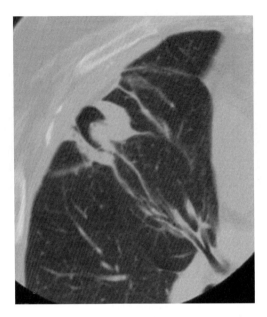

Figure 93

Findings: A single image from high-resolution CT of the chest showed a focal parenchymal abnormality with a pleural-based nodular opacity with central lucency and a curvilinear density extending centrally to the hilum. Associated pleural thickening with a calcified pleural plaque also was observed.

Diagnosis: Round atelectasis.

Discussion: Round atelectasis is a form of lung collapse that occurs in a juxtapleural location and is most commonly seen in patients with asbestos-related pleural disease. Its importance in recognition is that it can be confused with a pulmonary parenchymal mass. Round atelectasis also can form as a result of a pleural inflammation or infection, and thus is not solely related to asbestosis exposure. It is thought to arise initially as a focal area of atelectasis in the lung when a pleural effusion occurs as an inflammatory response to the offending asbestos fibers or other insult. As the effusion resolves, the lung becomes trapped, folded, and distorted as the surrounding lung reexpands.

Radiographically, the findings of round atelectasis are that of a juxtapleural masslike opacity, usually ranging in size from 2 to 5 cm, which has associated pleural thickening and a characteristic pattern of distortion of the vessels coursing into the involved segment of lung. The vessels are bunched together as they extend toward the hilum, but fan out around the area of involvement as they extend peripherally to the area of opacity in a characteristic "comet tail" appearance. The fanning out around the area also has been described as an appearance resembling the cords of a parachute.

Overall, when an area of round atelectasis is suspected, it should be followed to document stability over time, because round atelectasis should remain relatively unchanged over time, whereas a pulmonary parenchymal mass such as a bronchogenic carcinoma grows over time. If there is a question of the diagnosis, especially in a high-risk patient, than core biopsy may be helpful to exclude a malignancy.

CASE 94

History: A 29-year-old black man with a history of osteogenic sarcoma of the upper extremity had been treated extensively with chemotherapy and right upper extremity amputation, without improvement in the rapid progression of his disease.

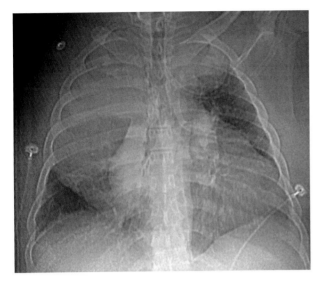

Figure 94A

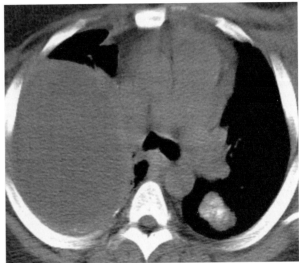

Figure 94B

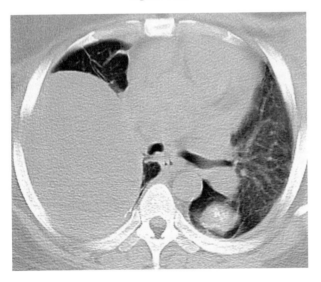

Figure 94C

Findings: A scout topographic image and CT of the chest in soft tissue and lung windows without contrast demonstrated a large, loculated, low-attenuation collection in the right upper hemithorax and left lung apex, as well as a partially calcified lung parenchymal mass in the left lower lobe. A pericardial effusion also was present.

Diagnosis: Metastases to the lung from osteosarcoma.

Discussion: Metastases from osteosarcoma and chondrosarcoma are two lesions that often contain calcifications. Other metastases that can contain calcifications include papillary carcinoma of the thyroid, ovarian carcinoma, and occasionally lung carcinoma following treatment with chemotherapy or radiation. Other metastatic lesions that can commonly show calcification include breast carcinoma, testicular cancer, and mucinous adenocarcinoma. Osteosarcoma metastases also may be associated with the presence of a pneumothorax.

Solitary or limited sarcomatous metastases to the lung are often surgically resected. Resection has been shown to prolong survival, although resection of the metastases is generally not anticipated to be curative.

CASE 95

History: A 48-year-old black woman with a history of end-stage renal disease is hemodialysis dependent secondary to hypertensive nephropathy. She also has a history of long-standing mitral valve disease and hypertensive cardiomyopathy. She was admitted with increasing shortness of breath and chest pain.

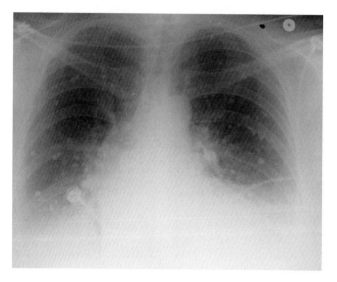

Figure 95

Findings: A single frontal radiographic view of the chest showed findings of chronic congestive failure, including bilateral pleural effusions and an enlarged heart. There was splaying of the carina from left atrial enlargement. Diffusely calcified nodular densities were seen throughout both lung fields.

Diagnosis: Diffuse ossification in the lungs from chronic congestive failure and mitral valve disease.

Discussion: Although very rare, occasionally diffuse pulmonary ossifications can be seen with long-standing mitral valve disease. These may show bony trabeculation histologically. They are otherwise difficult to distinguish from granulomatous calcifications. This patient had a long history of severe hypertension, end-stage renal disease, and mitral valve disease.

This patient died from myocardial infarction on this admission. Autopsy was performed and showed diffuse hemorrhagic changes in the lung from chronic congestive heart failure and evidence of hypertensive cardiomyopathy and myocardial infarction.

CASE 96

History: A 46-year-old man with a history of non-Hodgkin's lymphoma had undergone a matched, unrelated donor bone marrow transplant. He presented with respiratory distress and had no symptoms of fever, chills, night sweats, or cough. CT of the chest was subsequently performed.

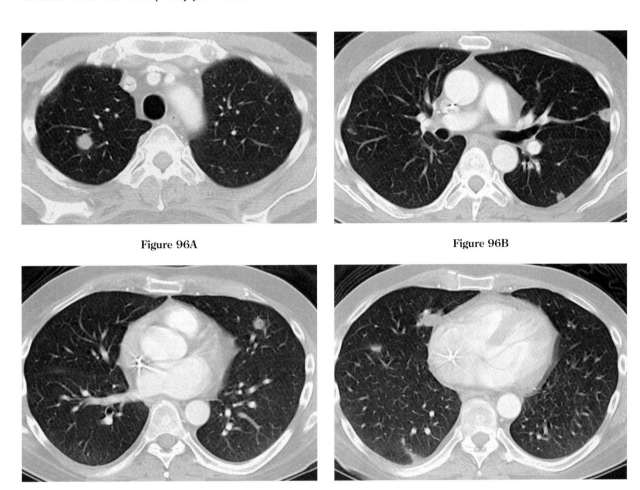

Figure 96A

Figure 96B

Figure 96C

Figure 96D

Findings: Four images from contrast-enhanced CT of the chest in lung windows demonstrated multiple small pulmonary parenchymal nodules, some of which had central cavitation. Some of the nodular areas of opacity were peripheral in location and somewhat wedge shaped.

Diagnosis: Aspergillosis.

Discussion: Infection with *Aspergillus fumigatus* is unusual in a host with a normal immune system, but is relatively common in immunocompromised patients, especially bone marrow transplant patients and patients being treated for lymphoma or leukemia. Patients may present radiographically with either a single or multiple areas of airspace opacity or with a diffuse tiny nodular or miliary pattern of involvement of the lungs. When multiple nodules are present, they often have irregular shaggy borders with indistinct margins. Air bronchograms also may be seen extending through the lesions.

Cavitation is not usually seen initially but can be seen as the nodular opacities evolve and as the host is able to mount an inflammatory response to the infection. Thus, a neutropenic patient may not show signs of cavitation within the lesions until he or she comes out of the neutropenic phase of treatment. On CT, a surrounding halo of ground-glass opacity may be seen around the lesions. This is a relatively characteristic appearance for *Aspergillus* infection, although it is not seen in all cases.

Associated hilar adenopathy is not usually seen with *Aspergillus* infection. Similarly, pleural effusions are not common, unless hemorrhagic infarction occurs.

SUGGESTED READING

Aberle DR, Gamsu G, Henschke CI, et al. A consensus statement of the Society of Thoracic Radiology: screening for lung cancer with helical computed tomography. *J Thorac Imaging* 2001;16:65–68.

Bonner JA. Non-small cell lung cancer. Introduction. *Semin Radiat Oncol* 2000;10:263–266.

Brant WE, Helms CA. *Fundamentals of diagnostic radiology,* 2nd ed. Philadelphia: Lippincott Williams & Wilkins, 1999:377–400.

Bungay HK, Davies RJ, Gleeson FV. CT scanning in lung cancer. *Thorax* 2001;56:84.

Cittadini G, Fiorini G, Giasotto V. Radiological assessment of clinical staging of lung cancer. *Ann Ital Chir* 1999;70:841–846.

Colby TV, Koss MN, Travis WD. Tumors of the lower respiratory tract. In: *Armed Forces Institute of Pathology Fascicle, Third Series.* Washington, DC: Armed Forces Institute of Pathology, 1995.

Dalrymple-Hay MJ, Drury NE. Screening for lung cancer. *J R Soc Med* 2001;94:2–5.

Diederich S, Wormanns D, Lenzen H, et al. Screening for asymptomatic early bronchogenic carcinoma with low dose CT of the chest. *Cancer* 2000;89(suppl):2483–2484.

Furrer M, Althaus U, Ris HB. Spontaneous pneumothorax from radiographically occult metastatic sarcoma. *Eur J Cardiothorac Surg* 1997; 11:1171–1173.

Haramati LB, White CS. MR imaging of lung cancer. *Magn Reson Imaging Clin North Am* 2000;8:43–57, viii.

Hasegawa M, Sone S, Takashima S, et al. Growth rate of small lung cancers detected on mass CT screening. *Br J Radiol* 2000;73: 1252–1259.

Henschke CI. CT/MR correlation in the evaluation of tracheobronchial neoplasia. *Radiol Clin North Am* 1990;28:555–571.

Jain P, Arroliga AC. Spiral CT for lung cancer screening: is it ready for prime time? *Cleve Clin J Med* 2001;68:74–81.

Klein JS, Webb WR. Radiologic staging of lung cancer. *J Thorac Imaging* 1991;7:29–47.

Lee KS, Shim YM, Han J, et al. Primary tumors and mediastinal lymph nodes after neoadjuvant concurrent chemoradiotherapy of lung cancer: serial CT findings with pathologic correlation. *J Comput Assist Tomogr* 2000;24:35–40.

Magne N, Porsin B, Pivot X, et al. Primary lung sarcomas: long survivors obtained with iterative complete surgery. *Lung Cancer* 2001;31: 241–245.

Medina JL. The value of transesophageal echography in the clinical staging of lung cancer. *Ann Ital Chir* 1999;70:847–849.

Meziane M, Decamp M. Low-dose spiral CT for lung cancer screening. *Cleve Clin J Med* 2001;68:84.

Miller YE. Staging of non-small-cell lung cancer with positron-emission tomography. *N Engl J Med* 2000;343:1571–1572; discussion 1572–1573.

Mintzer RA, Gore RM, Vogelzang RL, et al. Rounded atelectasis and its association with asbestos-induced pleural disease. *Radiology* 1981; 139: 567–570.

Munk PL, Muller NL, Miller RR, et al. Pulmonary lymphangitic carcinomatosis: CT and pathologic findings. *Radiology* 1988;166:705–709.

Naidich DP. Early lung cancer action project: overall design and findings from baseline screening. *Cancer* 2000;89(suppl):2474–2482.

Nenoff P, Kellermann S, Borte G, et al. Pulmonary nocardiosis with cutaneous involvement mimicking a metastasizing lung carcinoma in a patient with chronic myelogenous leukaemia. *Eur J Dermatol* 2000;10:47–51.

O'Donovan PB. The radiologic appearance of lung cancer. *Oncology (Huntington)* 1997;11:1387–1402; discussion 1402–1404.

Quinn D, Gianlupi A, Broste S. The changing radiologic presentation of bronchogenic carcinoma with reference to cell type. *Chest* 1996; 110:1474–147.

Solaini L, Bagioni P, Prusciano F, et al. Video-assisted thoracic surgery (VATS) lobectomy for typical bronchopulmonary carcinoid tumors. *Surg Endosc* 2000;14:1142–1145.

Tahara RW, Lackner RP, Graver LM. Is there a role for routine mediastinoscopy in patients with peripheral T1 lung cancers? *Am J Surg* 2000;180:488–492.

Takamochi K, Nagai K, Yoshida J, et al. The role of computed tomographic scanning in diagnosing mediastinal node involvement in non-small cell lung cancer. *J Thorac Cardiovasc Surg* 2000;119:1135–1140.

Tanaka F, Yanagihara K, Otake Y, et al. Biological features and preoperative evaluation of mediastinal nodal status in non-small cell lung cancer. *Ann Thorac Surg* 2000;70:1832–1838.

Tanoue LT. Pulmonary manifestations of rheumatoid arthritis. *Clin Chest Med* 1998;19:667–685, viii.

Tateishi U, Nishihara H, Watanabe S, et al. Tumor angiogenesis and dynamic CT in lung adenocarcinoma: radiologic-pathologic correlation. *J Comput Assist Tomogr* 2001;25:23–27.

Thompson BH, Stanford W. MR imaging of pulmonary and mediastinal malignancies. *Magn Reson Imaging Clin North Am* 2000;8:729–739.

Woodring JH. Pleural effusion is a cause of round atelectasis of the lung. *J Ky Med Assoc* 2000;98:527–532.

Yang ZG, Sone S, Li F, et al. Visibility of small peripheral lung cancers on chest radiographs: influence of densitometric parameters, CT values and tumour type. *Br J Radiol* 2001;74:32–41.

CHAPTER 6

HYPERLUCENT LUNG AND AIRWAYS

THOMAS DUNPHY
PATRICIA J. MERGO

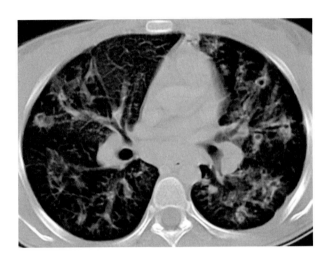

CASE 97

History: A 3-year-old with a history of asthma presented with increasing cough and fever of 2 weeks' duration.

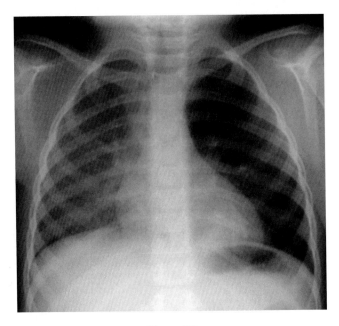

Figure 97

Findings: PA radiographic view of the chest demonstrated a hyperexpanded and hyperlucent left lung with minimal left lower lobe consolidation. The right lung was normal in appearance.

Differential Diagnosis: Airway obstruction from a foreign body in the left main bronchus with a postobstructive left lower lobe pneumonia should be considered.

Diagnosis: Foreign body (a Cheerio) in the left main bronchus with a postobstructive left lower lobe pneumonia.

Discussion: Aspiration of solid foreign bodies occurs most often in children. Fifty percent of cases occur in children under 3 years of age. The most commonly aspirated material is food, usually a vegetable or nut. A review of 160 patients who aspirated solid foreign bodies demonstrated that 85% aspirated vegetables, the most common being a peanut. The aspirated foreign body causes edema and inflammation with subsequent narrowing of the airway and air trapping. Distal atelectasis may occur acutely.

Chronic retention of a foreign body results in bronchial wall fibrosis and stenosis, usually accompanied by distal bronchiectasis and obstructive pneumonitis. The lower lobes are involved almost exclusively. There is no tendency toward one side or the other in children because the left and right bronchial angles are nearly equal up to the age of 15 years.

The radiographic findings are hyperexpansion of the ipsilateral lung due to air trapping. The affected lung is also hyperlucent due to hyperexpansion and oligemia from hypoxic vasoconstriction. These findings are best demonstrated on expiratory films, a decubitus film with the affected side down, or fluoroscopy. Fluoroscopy demonstrates air trapping in the ipsilateral lung and mediastinal swing of the heart to the contralateral side. Although not shown here, an expiratory film was obtained in this case and further demonstrated the findings of air trapping. Despite no history of a possible bout of aspiration, a foreign body was suspected. Bronchoscopy demonstrated a Cheerio in the left main bronchus with airway edema and inflammation.

CASE 98

History: The patient was a 35-year-old man with an abnormal chest radiograph and questionable pneumothorax.

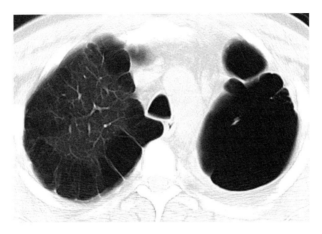

Figure 98A

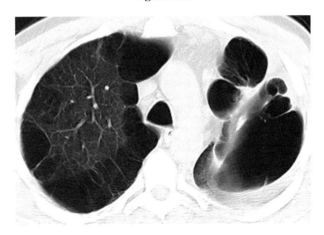

Figure 98B

Findings: Two images from CT of the chest in lung windows demonstrated extensive parenchymal lung destruction and bulla formation.

Diagnosis: Centrilobular bullous emphysema.

Discussion: Emphysema is defined as abnormal permanent enlargement of air spaces distal to the terminal bronchioles with destruction of alveolar walls and local elastic fiber network. The two major categories of emphysema are centrilobular and panacinar. Centrilobular emphysema is the most common form and is seen predominantly in the upper lung zones. Panacinar emphysema is seen predominantly in the lower lung zones and is best demonstrated in α_1-antitrypsin deficiency. Bullae are thin, septated, air-containing cystic spaces within lung parenchyma that are greater than 1 cm in diameter.

CASE 99

History: The patient was a 58-year-old smoker with COPD and increasing dyspnea and cough.

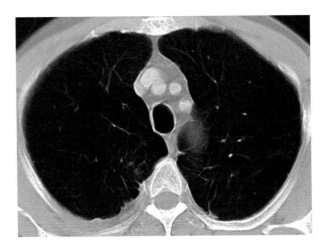

Figure 99

Findings: A CT image in lung windows demonstrated significant bilateral upper lobe parenchymal lung destruction consistent with emphysema.

Diagnosis: Centrilobular emphysema.

Discussion: Emphysema is an abnormal permanent enlargement of air spaces distal to the terminal bronchioles with destruction of alveolar walls and local elastic fiber network. The two major categories of emphysema are centrilobular (centriacinar) and panacinar. Other types of emphysema include periacinar (paraseptal) and cicatricial or scar emphysema. Centrilobular is the most common type of emphysema and is associated with destruction of parenchymal lung tissue in the region of the proximal respiratory bronchiole and alveoli. Centrilobular emphysema has upper zone predominance and is classically seen in smokers. It is also seen in coal workers.

Classic radiologic findings of emphysema are overinflation, oligemia, parenchymal lung destruction, and bulla formation. Associated findings include flattening of the hemidiaphragms and increase in the retrosternal air space, and a reduction in the size and number of pulmonary vessels, especially in the middle to outer portions of the lung. CT is helpful for further evaluating the extent of emphysema, and many recent studies suggest that CT quantification of the extent of involvement of the lung may provide a more accurate measure of lung function than pulmonary function tests by spirometry. Quantification with CT is achieved by measuring the amount of lung present that is of abnormal low attenuation as measured by Hounsefield units of less than -900 or -910.

CASE 100

History: A 45-year-old smoker presented with dyspnea that had increased over the preceding 2 years.

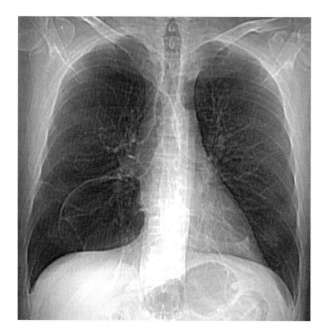

Figure 100A

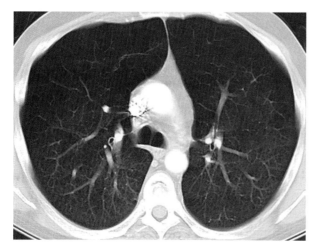

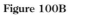

Figure 100B

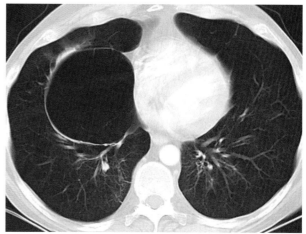

Figure 100C

Findings: A scout topographic image from CT of the chest demonstrated hyperexpansion of both lungs with oligemia and a single large bulla in the right lower lobe. CT images in lung windows demonstrated significant lung destruction predominantly in the bases, consistent with emphysema and a single large bulla in the right lower lobe.

Diagnosis: Panlobular emphysema secondary to α_1-antitrypsin deficiency.

Discussion: Emphysema is classically divided into two categories: centrilobular and panacinar. The centrilobular type is the most common form and has already been discussed (see Case 99). Panacinar emphysema consists of uniform, nonselective destruction of acini and secondary lobules. This form of emphysema has a lower lobe predilection and is associated with α_1-antitrypsin deficiency.

Alpha-1 antitrypsin is an acute phase reactant synthesized by the liver and released into the blood stream. This enzyme has a role in maintaining normal lung structure. Emphysema results from unchecked enzymatic destruction of the elastic and collagen framework of the lung. Deficiency of α_1-antitrypsin is associated with a 30-fold increase in the incidence of panacinar emphysema.

Smoking accelerates the rate of lung destruction; therefore, smokers with α_1-antitrypsin deficiency usually present in their third or fourth decade of life with symptoms of dyspnea. In comparison, nonsmokers with α_1-antitrypsin deficiency typically present in their fifth or sixth decade of life.

Radiographs typically demonstrate significant changes of emphysema with lung destruction, oligemia, hyperexpansion, and bulla formation primarily in the bases.

CASE 101

History: A 23-year-old woman was found to have an abnormal chest radiograph on routine physical examination for an advanced SCUBA certification evaluation.

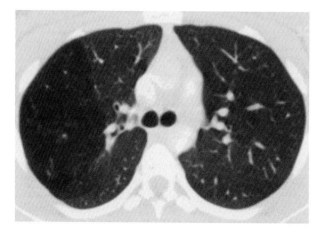

Figure 101A

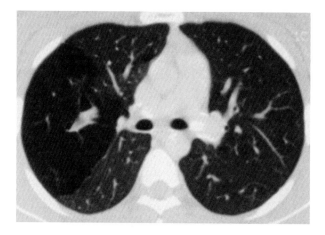

Figure 101B

Findings: Two views from CT of the chest demonstrated a segment of abnormal low attenuation of lung or hyperlucent lung in the right upper lobe. This area of low-density lung was hyperexpanded with an enlarged central tubular structure within it that contained an air-fluid level.

Differential Diagnosis: Airway obstruction from a foreign body or prior inflammatory process versus bronchial atresia should be considered.

Diagnosis: Bronchial atresia.

Discussion: The findings in this case demonstrate a hyperaerated segment of lung in the right upper lobe with a central dilated, mucous, and air-filled obstructed bronchus. This patient had bronchial atresia with no patent connection of the dilated bronchus to the more central tracheobronchial tree. Thus, mucous accumulated in the bronchus, causing it to dilate. The involved segment of lung became hyperexpanded because air entered the lung through the interstitium and the pores of Kohn, but the trapped air could not escape because its only means of escape was through the airway that was obstructed.

This patient's biggest point of concern was whether she could continue to SCUBA dive. She was instructed that the pressure changes that her lungs would undergo with SCUBA diving would put her at very high risk for pneumothorax; thus, she was advised against further SCUBA activity.

Bronchial atresia is uncommon and when seen usually involves the upper lobe apical or apicoposterior segments. The classic radiographic findings are similar to what is seen in this case, including a central masslike opacity that may have a tubular configuration or may contain an air-fluid level, which represents the dilated and obstructed bronchus distal to the point of obstruction, and hyperinflation of the involved segment of lung as described above. In addition, a relative paucity of vessels is evident in the involved segment of lung, because the vascular supply to the affected segment is obstructed or absent as well.

History: An 18-year-old college student presented to the emergency room with increasing cough; a note was made of the recent loss of her nose ring.

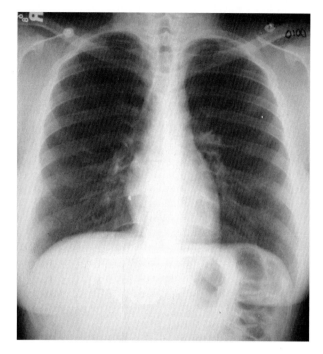

Figure 102A

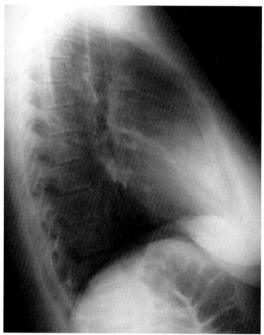

Figure 102B

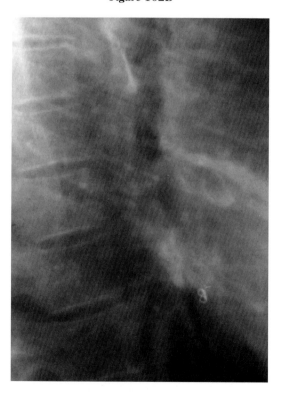

Figure 102C

Findings: PA and lateral chest radiographs and a close-up view of the lateral film demonstrated a metallic foreign body resembling the back of an earring projecting behind the heart on the lateral film and over the right aspect of the heart border on the PA view.

Diagnosis: Foreign body aspiration of the back of a nose ring.

Discussion: The patient's position and the bronchial anatomy are important factors in determining the distribution of the aspiration. In a supine patient, the posteriorly located segmental bronchi are frequent recipients of aspirated material. These bronchi go to the posterior segment of the right upper lobe, as well as the posterior basal and superior segments of the both lower lobes. This explains why these segments are most commonly affected by aspiration pneumonia. The right lung is more often involved than the left because the right main bronchus takeoff is straighter than that of the left main bronchus.

CASE 103

History: A 42-year-old man suffered a cardiac arrest while driving. The patient's car veered off the road and he was found unconscious at the scene. Emergency medical service personnel intubated the patient in the field.

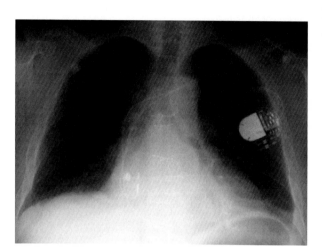

Figure 103A

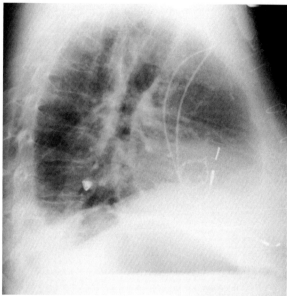

Figure 103B

Findings: PA and lateral chest radiographs demonstrated a dense foreign body in the shape of a tooth projecting over the right lower lobe. In addition, the heart was enlarged, with splaying of the carina from left atrial enlargement, and a pacing device was in place.

Diagnosis: Aspiration of a tooth into the posterior segment of the right lower lobe after intubation.

Discussion: Trauma during intubation can cause dislodgement of teeth. The aspirated teeth are often discovered on routine chest films. Overall, the most commonly aspirated foreign body is food, usually a nut or vegetable. Inhalation of foreign bodies is also much more common in children, especially in the first 3 years of life.

If the diagnosis is not recognized immediately or made within the first 2 to 3 days following the aspiration, then symptoms can often be prolonged and the diagnosis may not be made for weeks or months. Symptoms of a persistent cough or findings of a persistent area of atelectasis or pneumonia, especially in an impaired patient, should raise the suspicion of a possible foreign body aspiration. Only a minority of foreign bodies (<15%) are radiopaque enough to be seen on chest radiographs.

The foreign body incites an inflammatory reaction in the bronchus that can be severe and cause further obstruction as airway edema occurs. Peanuts are notorious for inciting a severe inflammatory response in the airways. If the foreign body is long-standing, then bronchiectasis of the involved segment of lung can result.

CASE 104

History: A 68-year-old man with a known history of squamous cell carcinoma of the esophagus developed fevers and shortness of breath shortly after starting radiation therapy.

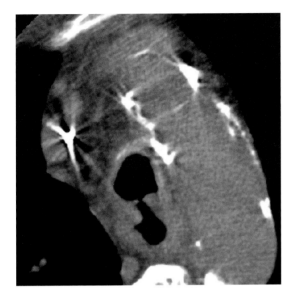

Figure 104A

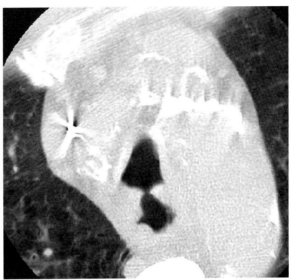

Figure 104B

Findings: Two cone-down images of the trachea from CT of the chest at the level of the aortic arch, in soft tissue and lung windows, demonstrated a fistulous connection between the trachea posteriorly and the esophagus anteriorly. The esophageal wall was diffusely thickened, and there was loss of the normal fat planes between the esophagus and the aortic arch.

Diagnosis: Tracheoesophageal (TE) fistula secondary to erosion of the wall of the esophagus and the trachea from the patient's esophageal cancer and subsequent radiation therapy.

Discussion: There are two types of TE fistulas: congenital and acquired. Congenital types are often found at birth and are associated with other abnormalities (VATER complex). The most common type of acquired TE fistula is due to esophageal cancer and is often precipitated by radiation therapy.

Other causes of TE fistulas include lymphoma, trauma, iatrogenic causes from intubation or endoscopic evaluation, corrosive esophagitis, and infection from histoplasmosis, tuberculosis or actinomycosis.

Once a TE fistula develops, the prognosis is extremely poor, with most patients dying within weeks to months. In patients being treated for malignancy who are felt to be at high risk for TE fistula development, an endoluminal stent can be placed prior to initiation of therapy to lessen the associated risk of morbidity and mortality.

CASE 105

History: A 13-year-old with a long history of a chronic illness presented with recurrent bouts of dyspnea and hemoptysis.

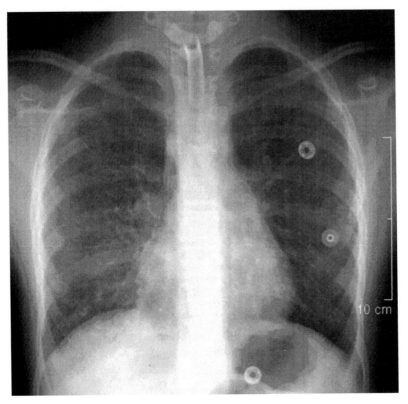

Figure 105

Findings: A PA radiographic view of the chest showed extensive cystic changes in the lower lung zones, particularly on the right. The cystic changes extended to the hilum. A tracheostomy tube was in place.

Diagnosis: Juvenile laryngeal papillomatosis.

Discussion: The papilloma is the most common benign tumor of the larynx and is caused by the human *Papillomavirus.* There is some debate as to whether there are two clinical forms, juvenile and adult. The adult form tends to be unifocal and easier to treat. Juvenile laryngeal papillomatosis is often multifocal and occurs in preschool children. Children usually present initially with hoarseness or stridor that may progress to dyspnea, dysphagia, pain, hemoptysis, cough, and respiratory distress. Two percent of patients develop involvement of the lower respiratory tract.

Radiographically, papillomas in the proximal bronchi can cause atelectasis and obstructive pneumonitis. Involvement of the distal airways can cause multiple nodular opacities that can cavitate. The dependent distal airways are typically involved as well because the papillomas spread through the tracheobronchial tree and are aerosolized during treatment.

CASE 106

History: A 25-year-old man with juvenile laryngeal papillomatosis was treated with biweekly bronchoscopy and carbon dioxide laser ablation. He had received a total of 256 treatments.

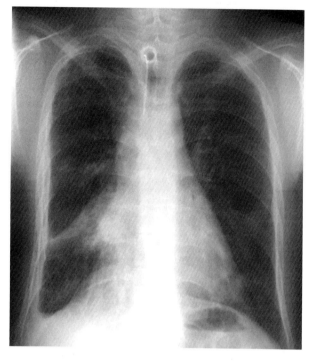

Figure 106A

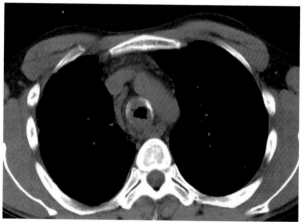

Figure 106B

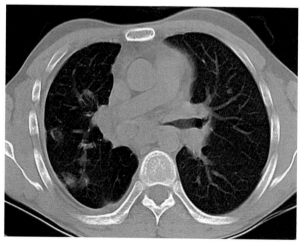

Figure 106C

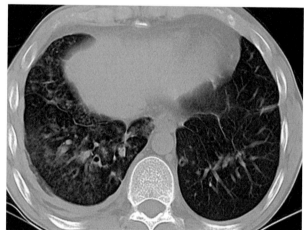

Figure 106D

Findings: A PA radiographic view of the chest demonstrated fluid in the minor fissure and a small right-sided pleural effusion. The lungs showed diffuse, scattered nodular opacities. A tracheostomy was in place. CT demonstrated irregular thickening and narrowing of the tracheal lumen. Lung parenchymal images at a lower level showed multiple nodular densities, primarily in the right lower lobe, and bronchiectasis and pleural thickening.

Differential diagnosis: Pneumonias (atypical bacterial, fungal, viral), tuberculosis, sarcoidosis, histiocystosis X, septic emboli, vasculitis, metastases, inhalational diseases, and juvenile laryngeal papillomatosis.

Diagnosis: Juvenile laryngeal papillomatosis.

Discussion: Treatment of laryngeal papillomatosis is controversial. Options include carbon dioxide laser, operative debridement, cryotherapy, argon laser after photosensitization, and systemic interferon therapy. There is some risk of malignant degeneration into squamous cell carcinoma. This patient had already undergone a partial right lower lobectomy for squamous cell carcinoma and presented as an extremely difficult case for management. His disease necessitated biweekly bronchoscopy and laser ablation therapy. Without the biweekly treatments, his trachea would rapidly narrow, resulting in respiratory compromise. At its most narrow portion, the trachea measured 6 mm in diameter. Tracheal stent placement had been considered, but had not yet been performed.

CASE 107

History: A 26-year-old chronically ill patient presented with nausea, vomiting, and dehydration.

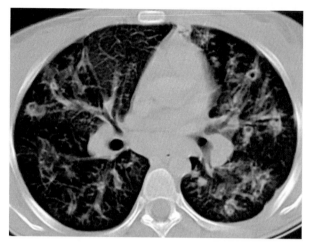

Figure 107A

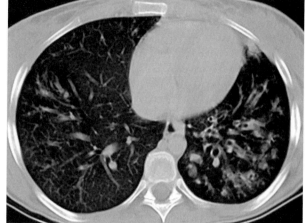

Figure 107B

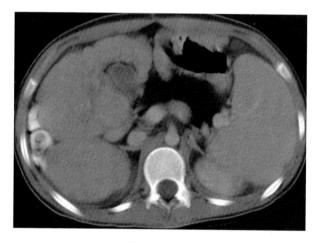

Figure 107C

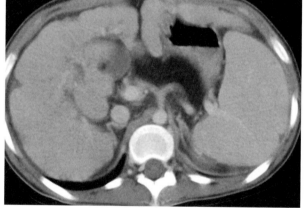

Figure 107D

Findings: CT images of the chest in lung windows demonstrated profound, diffuse, cystic dilatation of the airways. CT images of the upper abdomen in soft tissue windows demonstrated a nodular, cirrhotic-appearing liver, splenomegaly, and complete fatty replacement of the pancreas.

Diagnosis: Cystic fibrosis.

Discussion: Cystic fibrosis is a multisystem disease caused by dysfunction of exocrine glands that produce viscid secretions. It has autosomal-recessive inheritance and is the most common lethal inherited disease of whites. Cystic fibrosis has an incidence of 1 in 1,600 live births and an estimated carrier rate of 1 in 20. Diagnosis is usually made by a positive sweat test and appropriate clinical symptoms.

Pulmonary manifestations include chronic cough, recurrent pulmonary infections (with *Pseudomonas* colonization), and progressive respiratory insufficiency with development of cystic bronchiectasis.

Gastrointestinal manifestations include chronic obstipation, failure to thrive, meconium ileus in 10% to 15% of neonates, meconium ileus equivalent later in life, and jejunization of the colon. The liver is involved as well, with focal biliary cirrhosis from inspissated bile in 25% of patients, signs of portal hypertension, and hepatosplenomegaly. Inspissated pancreatic secretions are also seen with pancreatic insufficiency, steatorrhea, malabsorption of fats and protein, vitamin deficiency, diabetes mellitus, and fatty replacement of the pancreas. The paranasal sinuses also may be involved, with opacification of sinuses from recurrent sinusitis.

The prognosis of patients has improved over the years with antibiotic therapy. The mean life expectancy without lung transplantation is approximately 30 years. Ninety-five percent of patients die of respiratory insufficiency.

CASE 108

History: A 20-year-old chronically ill patient presented with dyspnea.

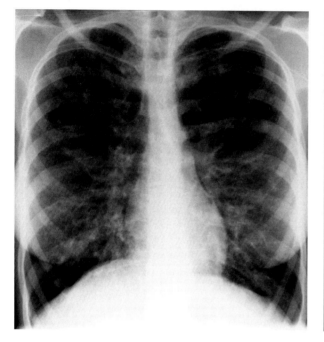

Figure 108A

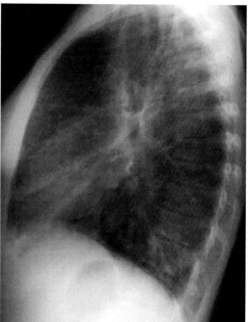

Figure 108B

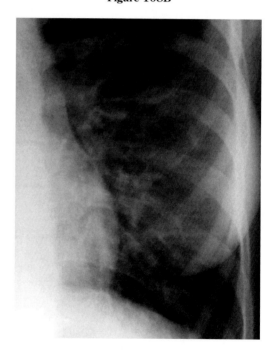

Figure 108C

Findings: PA and lateral radiographic views of the chest and a cone-down view of the PA chest demonstrated bilateral, predominately lower lobe bronchial wall thickening and dilatation.

Differential Diagnosis: Bronchiectasis caused by either cystic fibrosis, immune deficiency state, recurrent infection such as tuberculosis, or repeated allergic pneumonitis should be considered.

Diagnosis: Cystic fibrosis.

Discussion: Bronchiectasis is defined as irreversible abnormal dilatation of the bronchial tree. The most important mechanism is response to repeated infection. There are numerous causes of bronchiectasis, including congenital structural defects with abnormal collection of secretions (cystic fibrosis), immune deficiency states (immunoglobulin G deficiency), repeated infection (e.g., tuberculosis), bronchial obstruction (mucoid impaction), aspiration, and pulmonary fibrosis.

There are three classifications of bronchiectasis given in order of severity: cylindrical or tubular, varicose, and saccular/cystic. Cylindrical is the least severe type and consists of bronchi gradually becoming larger as they move distally. Varicose bronchiectasis involves a greater degree of dilatation, with focal constrictions resembling varicose veins. Saccular or cystic bronchiectasis is the most severe form, with progressive dilatation of the bronchial tree resulting in cystic spaces measuring up to several centimeters that may be filled with fluid.

Symptoms of bronchiectasis include cough, purulent sputum, dyspnea, and hemoptysis. The cause of hemoptysis is increased bronchial artery flow, which can be embolized percutaneously if necessary.

CASE 109

History: An 18-year-old nonsmoker presented with several bouts of hemoptysis.

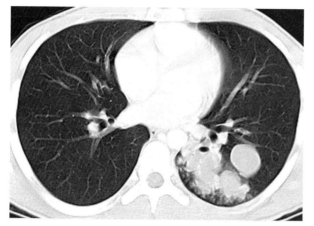

Figure 109A

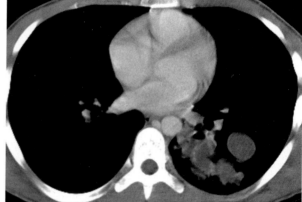

Figure 109B

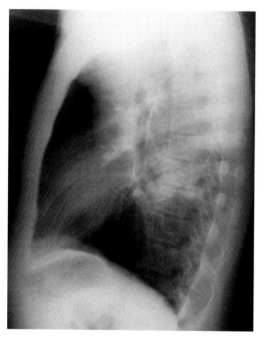

Figure 109C

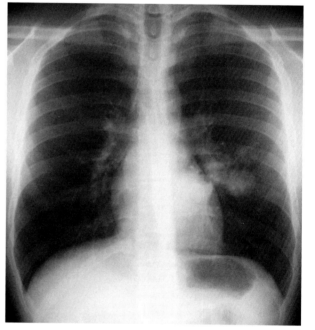

Figure 109D

Findings: PA and lateral radiographic views of the chest showed an elongated, tubular, finger-in-glove opacity in the left middle lung field. CT images in soft tissue and lung windows demonstrated round nodules in the left lower lobe with dilated, fluid-filled bronchi.

Differential Diagnosis: Mucoid impaction with associated saccular bronchiectasis or potential endobronchial tumor should be considered.

Diagnosis: Mucoid impaction with saccular bronchiectasis.

Discussion: Radiographic findings of bronchiectasis include prominent bronchial walls visible as parallel lines or single thickened lines. Ringlike opacities that may contain air-fluid levels are caused by thickened airway walls. Lung volumes may be increased with cystic fibrosis.

The definitive diagnosis of bronchiectasis is made by high-resolution CT. CT findings include thickened bronchial walls that may have a tram track or beaded appearance and bronchial dilatation. Bronchial dilatation is generally defined as a bronchial wall that is larger in diameter than the adjacent vessel. The signet ring sign is characteristic of a dilated bronchus next to its adjacent vessel in a cross-sectional imaging plane. When the dilated airway is seen along its longitudinal course, the tram track sign is more apparent.

Findings of cystic bronchiectasis include a "string of beads" appearance, continuity of the cystic structures with the airway, and the appearance of thick-walled cysts.

In this case, the patient had a long-standing mucoid impaction resulting in chronic obstruction of the distal airways in the left lower lobe and development of lobar saccular bronchiectasis.

SUGGESTED READING

Aubry MC, Wright JL, Myers JL. The pathology of smoking-related lung diseases. *Clin Chest Med* 2000;21:11–35, vii.

Bhalla M, Turcios N, Aponte V, et al. Cystic fibrosis: scoring system with thin-section CT. *Radiology* 1991;179:783–788.

Cheatham ML, Safcsak K. Air travel following traumatic pneumothorax: when is it safe? *Am Surg* 1999;65:1160–1164.

Cleveland RH, Neish AS, Zurakowski D, et al. Cystic fibrosis: predictors of accelerated decline and distribution of disease in 230 patients. *AJR Am J Roentgenol* 1998;171:1311–1315.

Erasmus JJ, McAdams HP, Farrell MA, et al. Pulmonary nontuberculous mycobacterial infection: radiologic manifestations. *Radiographics* 1999;19:1487–1505.

Espinola D, Rupani H, Camargo EE, et al. Ventilation-perfusion imaging in pulmonary papillomatosis. *J Nucl Med* 1981;22:975–977.

Greene KE, Takasugi JE, Godwin JD, et al. Radiographic changes in acute exacerbations of cystic fibrosis in adults: a pilot study. *AJR Am J Roentgenol* 1994;163:557–562.

Grenier P, Lenoir S, Brauner M. Computed tomographic assessment of bronchiectasis. *Semin Ultrasound CT MR* 1990;11:430–441.

Guest PJ, Hansell DM. High resolution computed tomography (HRCT) in emphysema associated with alpha-1-antitrypsin deficiency. *Clin Radiol* 1992;45:260–266.

Gurney JW. The pathophysiology of airways disease. *J Thorac Imaging* 1995;10:227–235.

Hansell DM. Bronchiectasis. *Radiol Clin North Am* 1998;36:107–128.

Hsu JT, Barrett CR. Unilateral hyperlucent lung. Patent ductus arteriosus coexisting with bronchial carcinoid. *Chest* 1979;76:325–327.

Kilburn KH, Warshaw RH, Thornton JC. Do radiographic criteria for emphysema predict physiologic impairment? *Chest* 1995;107:1225–1231.

Kuhlman JE, Reyes BL, Hruban RH, et al. Abnormal air-filled spaces in the lung. *Radiographics* 1993;13:47–75.

Maffessanti M, Candusso M, Brizzi F, et al. Cystic fibrosis in children: HRCT findings and distribution of disease. *J Thorac Imaging* 1996;11:27–38.

Morehead RS. Bronchiectasis in bone marrow transplantation. *Thorax* 1997;52:392–393.

Morishima M. The unilateral hyperlucent lung. *Nurse Pract* 1980;5:60–61.

Ruzal-Shapiro C. Cystic fibrosis. An overview. *Radiol Clin North Am* 1998;36:143–161.

Solomon D, Smith RR, Kashima HK, et al. Malignant transformation in non-irradiated recurrent respiratory papillomatosis. *Laryngoscope* 1985;95:900–904.

Tasker AD, Flower CD. Imaging the airways. Hemoptysis, bronchiectasis, and small airways disease. *Clin Chest Med* 1999;20:761–773, viii.

Webb WR. Radiology of obstructive pulmonary disease. *AJR Am J Roentgenol* 1997;169:637–647.

CHAPTER 7

MEDIASTINAL DISEASE

PATRICIA J. MERGO

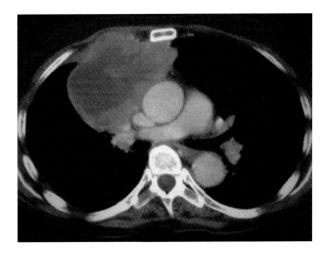

CASE 110

History: A 45-year-old woman had palpable enlargement of the right neck. CT was performed for further evaluation.

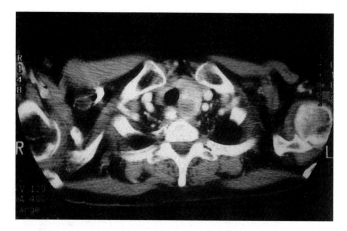

Figure 110

Findings: CT of the upper thorax demonstrated the mass high within the superior mediastinum in a left paratracheal location. The mass was overall low in attenuation and intimately associated with the thyroid gland on the left. The thyroid gland on the left was enlarged and had high density on this contrast-enhanced CT examination.

Diagnosis: Cystic thyroid goiter.

Discussion: The differential diagnosis for common anterior mediastinal masses is small. Four entities should be remembered, and they are prompted by the following mnemonic:

The Four T's

Thymoma
Teratoma
Thyroid mass
Terrible lymphoma

In terms of a more comprehensive discussion of anterior mediastinal masses, these entities can be grouped into cystic or solid lesions based on their pathologic and radiologic features. They can be further classified as either true cysts or cystic masses.

Substernal goiters comprise 10% of all mediastinal masses. Seventy-five percent of all substernal goiters are located in the anterior mediastinum. These are usually multinodular with hemorrhagic or necrotic regions, which give rise to the cystic appearance on imaging. In addition, goiter tends to displace other mediastinal structures such as the trachea and esophagus, which are often posteriorly displaced by large goiters. This can result in airway compromise. Onset is usually insidious.

In terms of imaging characteristics, goiters are usually lobulated in appearance and should have continuity with the thyroid gland and the neck, as this case demonstrates. They are more commonly seen on the right than the left. Areas that are cystic due to old hemorrhage or necrosis, as in this case, show low attenuation by CT, or decreased echogenicity by ultrasonography. Areas of more recent hemorrhage are of higher attenuation on CT. More solid areas within the goiter have high attenuation on CT, secondary to increased iodine content. Their diagnosis is easier to distinguish when the process is multinodular and bilateral. When there is a single nodule evident, histologic evaluation of the tissue via fine-needle aspiration is often helpful in cementing the diagnosis.

CASE 111

History: A 54-year-old man with a 30-year history of smoking presented with a 6-month history of increasing exertional dyspnea and a 3-month history of productive cough.

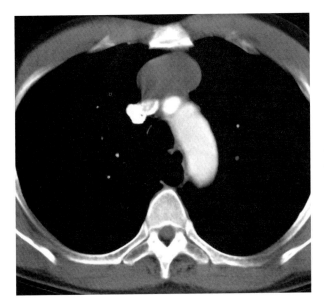

Figure 111A

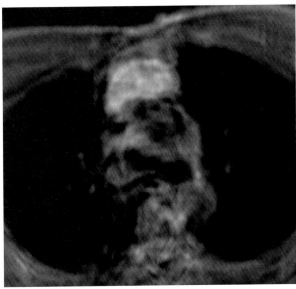

Figure 111B

Findings: CT showed a low-attenuation mass in the anterior mediastinum with the absence of additional mediastinal adenopathy. No calcifications were evident. MRI with T2 weighting demonstrated high-signal intensity of the mass consistent with fluid density.

Diagnosis: Thymic cyst.

Discussion: The differential diagnosis for anterior mediastinal masses seen on chest radiography include germ cell tumors, lymphoma, thyroid masses, and thymic tumors (i.e., the four T's). Cystic masses in the anterior mediastinum include two cysts such as pericardial cyst and thymic cyst, as well as cystic masses such as goiter, teratoma, lymphoma, or lymphangioma. This is a truly cystic mass, with the imaging findings of a simple cyst located contiguous with the thymus. Thymic cysts are rare and are usually congenital in origin, related to persistence of the thymopharyngeal duct. They are lined with either squamous or columnar cells. By imaging they are hypodense on CT and may be unilocular or multiloculated. They also may contain calcifications, although the lesion depicted in this case does not contain calcifications.

Key Imaging Findings of Thymic Cyst

Unilocular or multilocular
With or without calcifications
Hypodense

CASE 112

History: A 67-year-old woman with a 20-year history of tobacco use presented with a 1 year history of cough and a recent weight loss of 18 pounds. PA and lateral chest radiographs were obtained, with subsequent evaluation by CT.

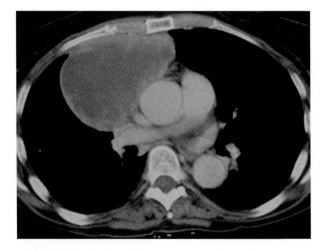

Figure 112A

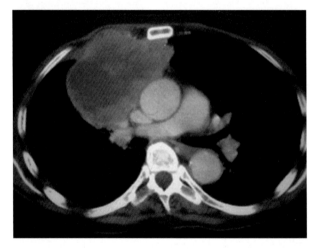

Figure 112B

Findings: Two images from a CT examination showed a mass in the anterior mediastinum. The mass had central low attenuation with peripheral enhancement. The line of demarcation from the adjacent mediastinal structures was not well defined. CT at a lower level demonstrated chest wall invasion into the right anterior chest wall. There was also right hilar adenopathy.

Diagnosis: Squamous cell carcinoma metastasis from lung carcinoma.

Discussion: By location and appearance this mass could easily represent that of either invasive thymoma, because there is chest wall invasion, or lymphoma. However, chest wall invasion is less likely seen with lymphoma. In this case, however, fine-needle aspirates demonstrated this to be squamous cell carcinoma with a presumed metastasis from a lung carcinoma primary tumor. Squamous cell carcinomas often have a cystic appearance, with central necrosis. Histologically, these tumors show central keratinization and yield a cystic appearance by imaging. Although many lesions can have this appearance by imaging, squamous cell carcinoma is a common lung neoplasm, as in this patient who has a long history of tobacco use.

CASE 113

History: A 10-year-old white girl presented with a history of cough on and off since birth. She had been treated with a variety of antibiotics multiple times in preceding years for bronchitis. In recent history, she presented with cough, fever and slightly decreased exercise tolerance. At this time a further evaluation was obtained. Radiographic imaging eventually led to MRI of the chest.

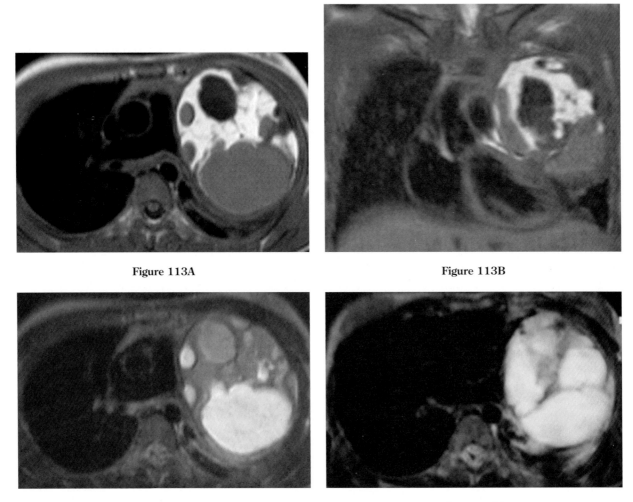

Figure 113A

Figure 113B

Figure 113C

Figure 113D

Findings: Axial and coronal T1-weighted MRI demonstrated a very large complex mass. The mass arose from the anterior mediastinum, although its origin was difficult to pinpoint secondary to its large size. The mass contained an area of high signal intensity on T1-weighted imaging secondary to fat evident within the lesion (A). There were also areas of low signal intensity, which were bright on T2-weighted imaging. Areas of intermediate signal intensity were observed on T1-weighted imaging, which were also noted to have intermediate signal intensity on T2-weighted imaging. A fat-suppression T1-weighted image (C) shows loss of signal in the fatty portions of the lesion; compare this to the conventional T1-weighted image (A). A T2-weighted axial image (D) demonstrated increased signal intensity within part of the mass, whereas areas that had increased signal intensity on T1-weighted imaging had low signal intensity on T2-weighted imaging.

Diagnosis: Anterior mediastinal teratoma.

Discussion: The differential diagnosis of an anterior mediastinal mass most commonly includes teratomas, thymomas, lymphomas, and thyroid lesions. Teratomas are usually seen as round or ovoid, smooth or lobulated masses in the superior or anterior mediastinum. They may contain two or three primitive cell derivatives. The mediastinum is the third most common location following a gonadal and sacrococcygeal origin. These lesions may be either benign or malignant. In general, mature (well-differentiated) teratomas are usually well-encapsulated and contain cystic components (either multilocular or unilocular). They may contain fat, bones (teeth), and hair. Malignant lesions account for approximately 30% of all teratomas and may have a more solid appearance.

These lesions are usually well circumscribed on cross-sectional imaging. On CT, calcifications are seen in approximately 25% of cases. Fatty and cystic elements result in low-density components on CT. Similarly, MRI may show areas of high signal intensity on T2-weighted imaging secondary to cystic components, and high signal intensity on T1-weighted imaging secondary to fatty components. It is difficult to distinguish between malignant lesions based on the imaging characteristics alone.

Germ cell tumors in general can have a cystic appearance within the mediastinum. The most common germ cell tumor, and the one most likely to be cystic, is teratoma. Other less common germ cell tumors include choriocarcinoma, seminoma, embryonal cell carcinoma and endodermal sinus tumor (yolk sac tumor), and mixed germ cell tumors. These tumors arise from primitive cell lines and are usually gonadal tumors. However, extragonadal germ cell tumors can occur, and when they do the mediastinum is a common location.

Choriocarcinomas have increased serum human chorionic gonadotropin levels, whereas embryonal cell carcinomas and yolk sac tumors are associated with elevated serum α-fetoprotein levels. In addition, choriocarcinomas are often hemorrhagic, which also may lead to a cystic appearance.

Key Imaging Findings of Teratoma

Smooth, lobulated surface, hair and/or teeth, calcifications in 25%
Cystic and solid components

CASE 114

History: This 47-year-old woman was asymptomatic, but findings were noted incidentally on a chest radiography performed as part of a routine physical examination.

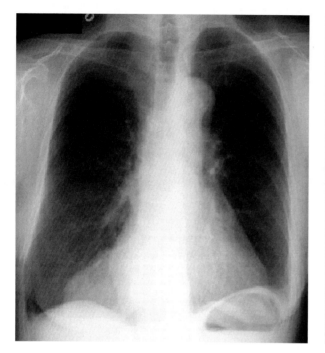

Figure 114A

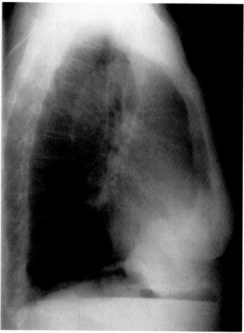

Figure 114B

Findings: PA and lateral chest radiographs showed a large density adjacent to the right heart border and projecting anteriorly on the lateral film. The masslike density was distinct from the adjacent cardiac silhouette.

Diagnosis: Pericardial cyst.

Discussion: Pericardial cysts are coelomic cysts that develop as a defect in embryologic development of the pleura or pericardium. They most commonly occur at the cardiophrenic angle, but because they are attached to the anterior aspect of the pericardium, and do not communicate with the pericardium, we will discuss them under the heading of anterior mediastinal masses. These cysts contain a mesothelial lining histologically.

By imaging, these cysts are distinguishable by their location (60% to 75% are located at the cardiophrenic angle) and by their low attenuation on CT, or corresponding very bright signal intensity on MRI. They do not usually contain calcifications. Another feature is their frequent mobility, as evidenced by changes in location with alterations in patient positioning.

Key Imaging Findings of Pericardial Cyst

60% to 75% at right cardiophrenic angle
Smooth margins
Low density
Unilocular
Isolated from pericardial sac

CASE 115

History: A 22-year-old man with a 6-month history of back and chest pain was treated at an outpatient clinic with pain medications for possible muscle strain. He presented recently with gastrointestinal distress, and after chest radiography showed an anterior mediastinal mass, he was admitted for further workup.

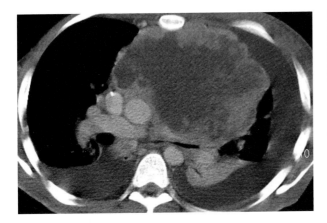

Figure 115A

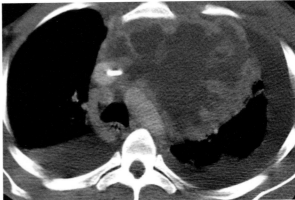

Figure 115B

Findings: Two images from a contrast-enhanced CT of the chest showed a large anterior mediastinal mass, with central low attenuation from necrosis and peripheral enhancement evident. The mass invaded the chest wall anteriorly and compressed the mediastinal structures posteriorly. Bilateral pleural effusions also were noted.

Diagnosis: High-grade B-cell non-Hodgkin's lymphoma with suggestive features of Burkitt's lymphoma.

Discussion: Lymphoma, generally thought of as a solid neoplasm, is cystic in 20% to 50% of cases. Anterior mediastinal involvement is more characteristic of Hodgkin's lymphoma (nodular sclerosing) than non-Hodgkin's lymphoma. Ninety percent of Hodgkin's lymphoma cases involve the anterior mediastinum, whereas 40% involve the anterior mediastinum only.

Imaging characteristics are that of a soft tissue mass, with cystic or low attenuation components in 20% to 50%, secondary to necrosis. Little enhancement is seen following intravenous contrast material administration (or gadolinium administration with MRI). Calcifications are not seen *de novo,* but are a frequent finding following treatment.

Key Imaging Findings of Lymphoma

Cystic in 20% to 50% (necrosis)
Little enhancement
May calcify after treatment

History: A 60-year-old woman was in her usual state of good health until she experienced an insidious onset of right-sided chest discomfort. She had no history of fever, chills, night sweats, cough, or hemoptysis. She was a nonsmoker. Chest radiography was subsequently performed. She had been hypothyroid since the age of 13 and treated medically with thyroid supplements.

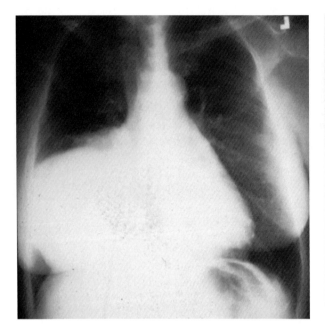

Figure 116A

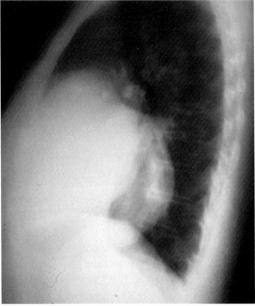

Figure 116B

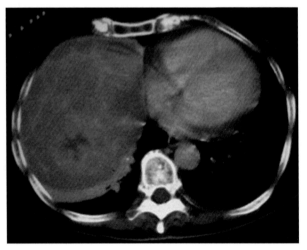

Figure 116C

Findings: PA and lateral chest radiographs demonstrated a large anteriorly located mass within the chest. This mass consumed much of the right lower hemothorax, and the margins were indistinguishable from that of the cardiac silhouette on the right. The mass did have a distinct demarcation on the lateral film from the cardiac silhouette and projected to opacify the entire anterior costophrenic angle. CT demonstrated a large mass within the right hemithorax, which was adjacent to the cardiac silhouette. There appeared to be preservation of the epicardial fat. The mass had a heterogeneous appearance with areas of contrast enhancement within it. There was a more central area of decreased attenuation, which was a cystic component of the mass. Posteriorly there was atelectatic lung, which was adjacent to the mass.

Diagnosis: Invasive thymoma.

Discussion: Thymoma is the most common primary mediastinal tumor. Both noninvasive and invasive forms exist, with 70% of lesions being benign. Thirty percent of thymoma patients have myasthenia gravis (remember: 30 thymomas), whereas only 15% of myasthenia gravis patients have thymoma. There are other associations, in addition to myasthenia gravis, including aplastic anemia, Cushing's disease, and hypogammaglobulinemia. Thymomas are characterized by a proliferation of lymphoid and epithelial cells, surrounded by a fibrous capsule. Histologically, the cells do not have a malignant morphology, but the tumor can be invasive. The invasive form tends to invade lobular structures and most commonly spreads to the pleura or pericardium. Thymomas can contain cysts microscopically or grossly, but are only cystic in appearance by imaging in approximately 5% of cases. Other imaging features include that of a well-circumscribed, lobulated, homogeneous mass of soft tissue attenuation on CT. Calcifications are evident in approximately 25%. Although it is impossible to distinguish benign from invasive thymomas by imaging findings alone, the involvement of adjacent structures or the presence of associated pleural or pericardial thickening are indicators of more invasive disease.

Key Imaging Findings of Thymoma

Base of heart
Well-demarcated
CA^{2+} in up to 25%
5% cystic

CASE 117

History: A 76-year-old man originally presented 3 years earlier with hypernasal speech, bilateral ptosis, and nasopharyngeal regurgitation with swallowing. He had reported some dysphagia and neck weakness at that time, which increased over the 3-year interval. Workup at that time with CT of the chest demonstrated the following findings.

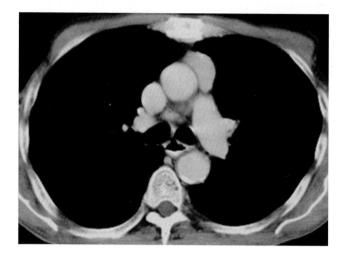

Figure 117

Findings: A single image from contrast-enhanced CT demonstrated a solid, homogenous, enhancing mass in the anterior mediastinum, which was well-demarcated from the ascending aorta and other mediastinal structures. This mass had a lobulated, well-circumscribed appearance.

Diagnosis: Thymoma in a patient with myasthenia gravis.

Discussion: At this patient's initial time of evaluation, he had a positive Tensilon test result with acetylcholine receptor antibody positivity. These findings led to an initial diagnosis of myasthenia gravis. The patient also had an anterior mediastinal mass, which was confirmed to be a thymoma. Thirty percent of thymoma patients have myasthenia gravis, whereas only 15% of myasthenic patients have thymoma. This mass had a more solid appearance typical of thymomas and was well-circumscribed. It is difficult to tell invasive from noninvasive thymomas based on imaging characteristics alone. When there is obvious chest wall invasion, this becomes more easily distinguishable by imaging. This case demonstrates the imaging appearance of a well-circumscribed, lobulated homogeneous mass of soft tissue attenuation. Note that this example does not demonstrate dense calcifications, which are seen in approximately 25% of cases. However, there is a very small area of increased attenuation within the anterior aspect of the mass, which probably represents a small calcification.

CASE 118

History: An 88-year-old woman with a history of dementia of the Alzheimer type fell and fractured her proximal left humerus. She was brought to the emergency room for further treatment. Chest radiography on admission demonstrated a large calcified mass in the anterior superior mediastinum.

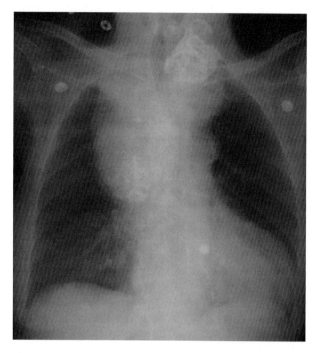

Figure 118A

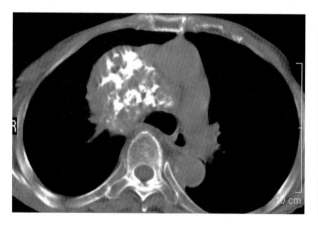

Figure 118B

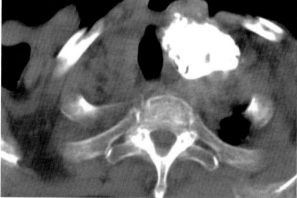

Figure 118C

Findings: A PA chest radiograph demonstrated a large mediastinal mass that contained extensive calcifications and extended up into the neck. There was deviation of the trachea and proximal right main bronchus as well. Two CT images showed a densely calcified mass. Dense calcification was seen in the left neck. At a lower level, the mass assumed a right peritracheal location, displacing the trachea and aorta toward the left. There were very coarse, dense calcifications within this well-circumscribed mass.

Diagnosis: Thyroid goiter.

Discussion: This case illustrates a grand champion thyroid goiter in this relatively asymptomatic 88-year-old woman. The imaging features are characteristic of thyroid goiter with continuity with the thyroid gland, dense calcifications seen within the lesion, and displacement of the trachea and other mediastinal structures. There was no real airway compromise, although this could become apparent with a further increase in size. This lesion does not contain cystic components, but has a more solid appearance.

Key Imaging Findings for Substernal Goiter

1. Continuity with the thyroid gland
2. High attenuation on CT
3. Trachea deviation
4. Focal Ca^{2+}
5. Cystic areas

CASE 119

History: A 38-year-old white woman had been in excellent health until she discovered a lump in her left lower cervical region. A 6-cm palpable neck mass was evident on physical examination. CT of the chest was subsequently performed.

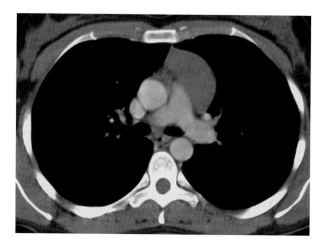

Figure 119

Findings: A single image from contrast-enhanced CT of the chest showed a solid homogenous mass in the anterior mediastinum. The remainder of the mediastinum was not involved with significant adenopathy, and examination of the abdomen and pelvis similarly showed no evidence of disease. Thus, the imaging findings were limited to a solid anterior mediastinal mass.

Diagnosis: Hodgkin's lymphoma.

Discussion: Hodgkin's lymphoma can be divided into four subtypes, including nodular sclerosing Hodgkin's lymphoma and three additional subtypes, which are based on the proportion of Sternberg-Reed giant cells present and include lymphocyte-predominant, mixed cell, and lymphocyte-depleted classifications. The lymphocyte-depleted subtype has the worst prognosis overall.

Most patients present in their second or third decade of life, although there is a second peak in the fifth and sixth decade of life. As in this case, an initial presentation with cervical adenopathy is commonly encountered. Other symptoms can include fever, night sweats, fatigue, weight loss, anorexia, and occasionally pruritus.

Staging classification of Hodgkin's disease includes four stages. Stage I disease has involvement of a single organ or lymph node region. Stage II disease involves two or more lymph node regions on the ipsilateral side of the diaphragm. Stage III disease involves lymph nodes on both sides of the diaphragm, and there may be involvement of the spleen or other localized organ involvement. Finally, stage IV disease is characterized by diffuse involvement of one or more extralymphatic organs.

Anterior mediastinal and paratracheal adenopathy are the most common sites of involvement with Hodgkin's disease. Nodular sclerosis Hodgkin's disease in particular has a propensity for anterior mediastinal involvement. Subcarinal involvement also can be seen, but isolated hilar adenopathy or posterior mediastinal adenopathy is uncommon with Hodgkin's lymphoma.

CASE 120

History: A 49-year-old man with a history of hypertension presented with worsening chest pain, dyspnea, and neck swelling over a 1-week period. He had a prior history of positive PPD with INH therapy for 1 year. He also had a history of smoking approximately half a pack of cigarettes per day and drinking 1 to 2 pints of alcohol per week.

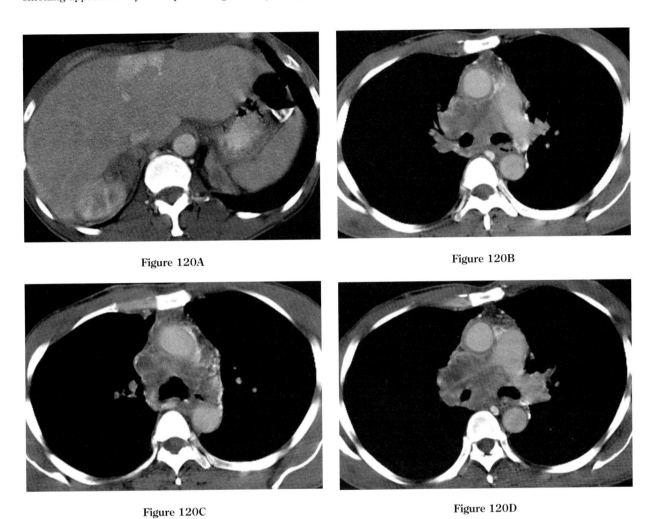

Figure 120A

Figure 120B

Figure 120C

Figure 120D

Findings: CT demonstrated extensive predominantly middle mediastinal adenopathy, with some posterior and anterior mediastinal involvement. The superior vena cava was occluded. Contrast partially filled the superior vena cava with a definite filling defect present within the superior vena cava and left subclavian vein. At a lower level, the right upper lobe bronchus was narrowed with a peripheral pulmonary parenchymal nodule. There was central hilar and mediastinal adenopathy, which encroached upon the pulmonary artery in addition to the superior vena cava. CT through the upper abdomen demonstrated increased enhancement in the quadrate lobe of the liver (*A*). These findings are consistent with superior vena cava obstruction with collateralization of flow through the anterior abdominal wall, through the liver, and into the inferior vena cava.

Diagnosis: Superior vena cava obstruction from non–small cell carcinoma of the lung.

Discussion: As previously discussed, superior vena caval obstruction can occur as a result of extensive compression from a mass or from an actual clot within the superior vena cava itself. In this case, there was obstruction of the superior vena cava by extensive mediastinal adenopathy related to the patient's non–small cell carcinoma. Because of the obstruction, there was propagation of the clot proximally. Although this patient's history of a positive PPD and drug abuse might suggest an infectious etiology such as tuberculosis, histologic examination confirmed the presence of non–small cell lung carcinoma.

CASE 121

History: A 32-year-old woman presented with new onset of head and neck swelling.

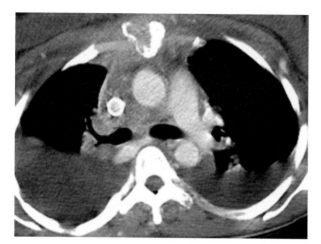

Figure 121A

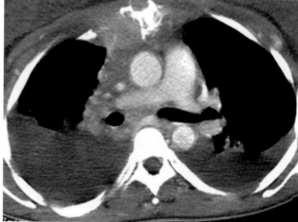

Figure 121B

Findings: CT showed a diffuse infiltrating soft-tissue density within the anterior and middle mediastinum with associated bilateral pleural effusions. A stent was placed in the superior vena cava with no contrast visible within the stent.

Computed tomography at a lower level demonstrated multiple collateral vessels along the anterior upper abdominal wall surface. In addition, there was increased enhancement within the quadrate lobe of the liver.

Diagnosis: Hodgkin's lymphoma with superior vena cava obstruction related to an infected infusiport.

Discussion: An infusiport had been placed in this patient for chemotherapy for Hodgkin's lymphoma. She subsequently developed superior vena cava obstruction, and a stent was placed into the superior vena cava. The lack of contrast enhancement of the superior vena cava and the stent, as well as the increased collateral vessels in the anterior abdominal wall and quadrate lobe of the liver, confirmed the persistence of superior vena cava obstruction. With superior vena cava obstruction, collateral vessels fill through the chest wall and the anterior abdominal wall into the inferior vena cava through the quadrate lobe of the liver. Superior vena cava obstruction can be iatrogenic in nature, or can be secondary to extrinsic compression from tumor or direct involvement from tumor extension.

CASE 122

History: A 33-year-old woman was noted to have an abnormal chest radiograph as part of a routine physical examination.

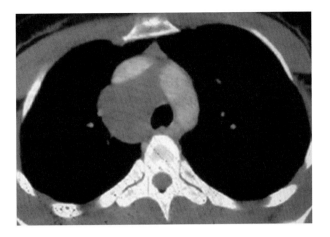

Figure 122

Findings: A single image from contrast-enhanced CT of the chest showed a large (5 cm), low-attenuation, smoothly contoured mass in a right paratracheal location. This mass involved the middle and posterior mediastinum and had an imperceptibly thin wall with no calcifications or enhancement. It displaced the superior vena cava anteriorly. A normal triangular thymus was also visible in a retrosternal location, just anterior and to the left of the superior vena cava.

Diagnosis: Bronchogenic cyst.

Discussion:

Cystic Middle Mediastinal Masses

True Cysts

True cysts of the middle mediastinum include pericardial cysts, which were previously discussed, and bronchogenic and esophageal duplication cysts. Esophageal duplication cysts are more commonly encountered in the posterior mediastinum.

Bronchogenic Cysts

Bronchogenic cysts are a type of foregut cyst, resulting from abnormal budding or branching of the tracheobronchial tree. Although the most common site is within the lung parenchyma (lower lobes), they also can occur within the mediastinum (posterior and middle mediastinum most commonly). Most are located near the carina, with the subcarinal region being a particularly prevalent location. Histologically, bronchogenic cysts are lined with respiratory epithelium. The characteristic histologic feature is the presence of cartilage within the wall of the cyst. When located in the mediastinum, these cysts rarely communicate with the tracheobronchial tree.

Plain film radiographic features are that of a mediastinal mass (often subcarinal) that is smooth or rounded in contour. On cross-sectional imaging, they are well-defined masses of low attenuation on CT. Calcifications are usually not present. On MRI, the high water content of the cysts yields very bright signal intensity on T2 weighted image.

Key Imaging Features of Bronchogenic Cysts
Smooth contour
No calcium
Low attenuation
No connection with bronchial tree

CASE 123

History: An 81-year-old woman had undergone surgery for mesenteric ischemia. She had had a central line placed aberrantly for hemodialysis, and an undetermined amount of fluid was infused through the catheter. CT of the chest was obtained as a follow-up examination.

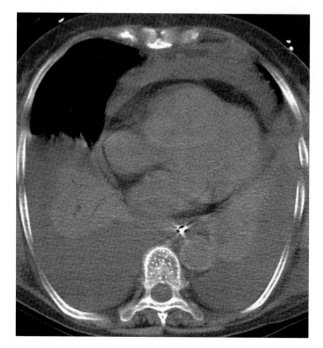

Figure 123A

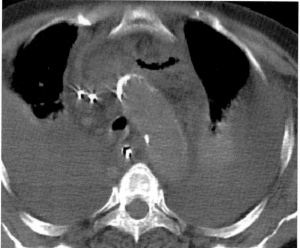

Figure 123B

Findings: Contrast-enhanced CT showed a large amount of low-attenuation material/fluid in the anterior and middle mediastinum. In addition, gas was present in the anterior mediastinum. There were also large bilateral pleural effusions and a large pericardial effusion.

Diagnosis: Mediastinitis.

Discussion: Acute mediastinitis is uncommon and is seen most often postoperatively following median sternotomy or another intervention such as line placement, or following perforation of the esophagus. The clinical presentation is usually that of a very sick patient with fevers, chills, and chest pain. The morbidity of mediastinitis is reported as being very high in the literature, but improved antibiotic therapy and advancement in percutaneous drainage techniques has somewhat lessened the associated mortality.

Radiographic findings include a widened mediastinum and pneumomediastinum. The air within the mediastinum may be difficult to appreciate on plain film radiographically, but is readily apparent by CT. Other CT findings include either diffuse infiltration of the mediastinum with a "dirty fat" appearance and loss of the normal fat planes or a localized fluid collection or abscess within the mediastinum.

It is often difficult to distinguish normal postoperative changes in the mediastinum following median sternotomy from infection, because some retrosternal air can be seen after surgery, as well as stranding of the mediastinal fat and obliteration of the normal fat planes. The postsurgical changes in the mediastinum can persist for up to 2 months, and residual air can be present for several weeks. Therefore, cementing the diagnosis of mediastinitis often depends on an appreciation of worsening of the findings on serial examinations, rather than on the findings of a single postoperative examination itself.

CASE 124

History: The patient was a 46-year-old man with a 30 pack-year history of smoking and a recent history of weight loss and hemoptysis.

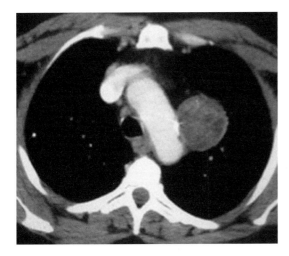

Figure 124A

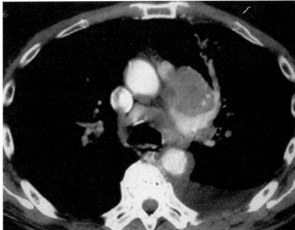

Figure 124B

Findings: Contrast-enhanced CT of the chest showed a 5-cm heterogenous, enhancing, low-attenuation mass involving the AP window and extending anteriorly up to the aorta. There was an associated mass effect and compression on the left pulmonary artery by the mass.

Diagnosis: Metastases from small cell carcinoma.

Discussion: Any metastasis to the middle mediastinum, which is necrotic in nature, may have a cystic appearance on cross-sectional imaging. Commonly encountered necrotic or cavitating metastases include squamous cell carcinoma (from lung carcinoma or from caudal extension from a neck primary tumor), sarcomatous metastases, and melanoma. Other primary bronchogenic carcinomas also can have a cystic appearance, although squamous cell carcinomas are the most common with this appearance secondary to their formation of keratin pearls.

This lesion is at risk for erosion into the left pulmonary artery by proximity. A lesion with this appearance may be mistaken for an aneurysm, arising either from the aorta or the pulmonary artery. However, its heterogenous appearance and internal enhancement allow this distinction to be made easily in this case. In less clear cases, however, CT or MR angiographic examination with dynamic arterial phase imaging usually can make this distinction readily.

CASE 125

History: The patient was a 74-year-old man with a history of known mediastinal adenopathy who underwent CT of the chest as part of a follow-up examination.

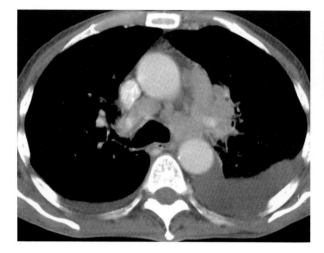

Figure 125A

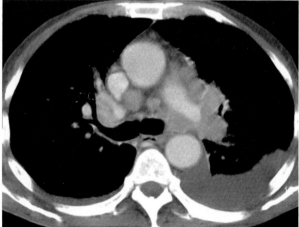

Figure 125B

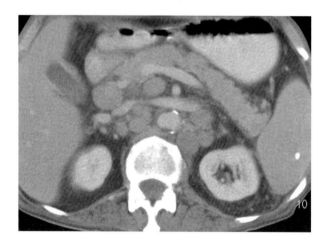

Figure 125C

Findings: CT of the chest and upper abdomen showed extensive adenopathy involving the middle mediastinum, left hilum, and AP window, as well as the retroperitoneum. The adenopathy compressed the left pulmonary artery and uplifted and surrounded the abdominal aorta. There also was an associated left pleural effusion.

Diagnosis: Angioimmunoblastic lymphadenopathy (AILD).

Discussion: Most solid middle mediastinal masses are attributable to lymphadenopathy, from either a neoplastic, infectious, or inflammatory etiology. Lymphomatous involvement can be from either Hodgkin's or non-Hodgkin's disease, with a 2:1 predominance, respectively.

AILD is an uncommon lymphoproliferative T cell disorder with generalized lymphadenopathy, rash, fever, hepatosplenomegaly, weight loss, and a polyclonal gammopathy. Two forms exist, including a benign form and AILD-type T-cell lymphoma. AILD usually affects patients in the seventh decade of life or older with onset of generalized lymphadenopathy, hepatosplenomegaly, fever, and weight loss. Forty percent of patients have a pruritic generalized rash, which may present as an exanthematous rash, purpura, generalized petechiae, bullous lesions, or acute lupus erythematous-like lesions. Mediastinal and abdominal adenopathy can be seen with imaging, which is indistinguishable from lymphoma. Systemic corticosteroids are often the first line of treatment and can lead to complete remission in 50% of patients. Despite treatment, the prognosis of AILD T-cell lymphoma is generally poor, with the mean survival period being less than 20 months.

CASE 126

History: A 50-year-old white woman with a 4-year history of asthma presented with worsened symptoms of dyspnea on exertion. The patient reported a nonproductive cough with exertion and exacerbated by environmental triggers.

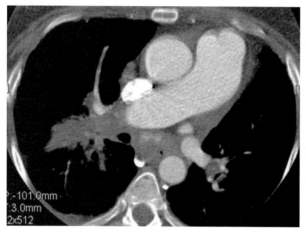

Figure 126A

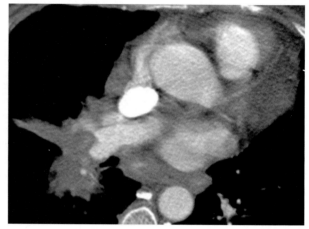

Figure 126B

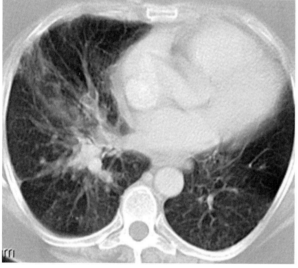

Figure 126C

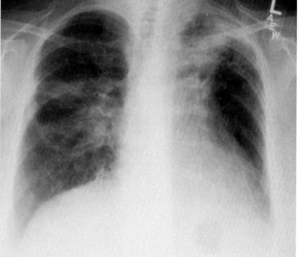

Figure 126D

Findings: A PA radiograph of the chest showed widening of the mediastinum with bilateral calcified hilar adenopathy. There was associated retraction of the hilum downward on the right and extensive fibrosis in the left upper lobe. CT of the chest with contrast showed extensive abnormal soft tissue density within the mediastinum, extending out into the central peribronchial interstitium with mass effect and extrinsic compression on the central pulmonary veins. There also were calcifications evident within the mediastinum. Lung parenchymal windows showed central peribronchial interstitial involvement with some interstitial nodules.

Diagnosis: Fibrosing mediastinitis.

Discussion: Fibrosing mediastinitis occurs as a rare complication of infection with *Histoplasma capsulatum*. With this process, invasion of adjacent normal structures, including mediastinal vessels and airways, by fibrous material occurs over long periods of time and may result in airway or vessel obliteration. It occurs most commonly in the third to fifth decade of life, and patients present most commonly with hemoptysis, with other symptoms including dyspnea, cough, and wheezing. Patients also may present with pulmonary edema from obstruction and obliteration of pulmonary venous return.

The most common radiographic findings in patients with fibrosing mediastinitis are mediastinal masses and parenchymal infiltrates. On occasion, however, the chest radiograph can be normal.

Computed tomography is helpful for further delineation of mediastinal involvement, with findings including obliteration of fat planes with abnormal soft tissue within the mediastinum, with or without the presence of a discrete mass. Treatment is supportive, with no effective therapy available. Antiinflammatory treatment with steroids has not been shown to be helpful, and surgical intervention is also not effective. Overall, the mortality rate for mediastinal fibrosis approaches 30%, with death ensuing from cor pulmonale or respiratory failure.

CASE 127

History: A 76-year-old woman originally presented with a right thigh mass. She was seen by an orthopaedist and diagnosed with bursitis for which she received injections in both her left hip and left knee, which did not alleviate the pain. She also had some sweating and fevers, but no other major problems. A follow-up evaluation revealed the diagnosis for which she was treated.

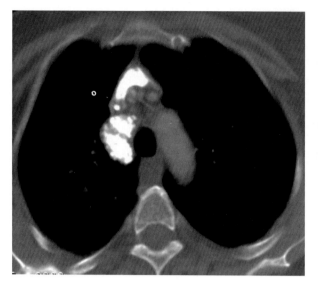

Figure 127A

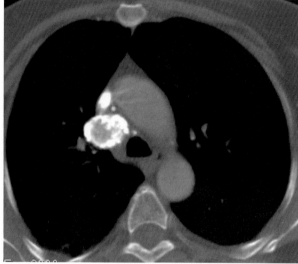

Figure 127B

Findings: Two images from a contrast-enhanced CT of the chest show densely calcified right paratracheal adenopathy. No other adenopathy was evident within the mediastinum or elsewhere at this time. The superior vena cava and left brachiocephalic vein are also densely opacified with iodinated contrast material.

Diagnosis: Calcified treated intermediate-grade large cell lymphoma of B-cell type.

Discussion: Calcified lymph nodes in the mediastinum can be seen with sarcoidosis, silicosis, coal worker's pneumoconiosis, and treated lymphoma, as well as with tuberculosis, histoplasmosis, or coccidioidomycosis. Any of the above mentioned processes can have peripheral egg shell type calcifications evident. This case, however, demonstrates diffuse dense calcifications, which also can be seen with any of the above mentioned entities.

Lymph node calcifications in patients with untreated lymphoma are very rare. Treated disease, however, can have diffuse calcifications, as in this case, or egg shell type or irregular calcifications. The calcified lymph nodes are difficult to distinguish from granulomatous calcifications, although the calcified lymph nodes may be larger than that typically seen with granulomatous disease. The given history of prior lymphoma, however, enables this distinction to be made.

CASE 128

History: A 35-year-old man collapsed while he was playing baseball when he was 5 years old. He was subsequently diagnosed as having a ventricular septal defect (VSD). He limited his activities during childhood and early adulthood.

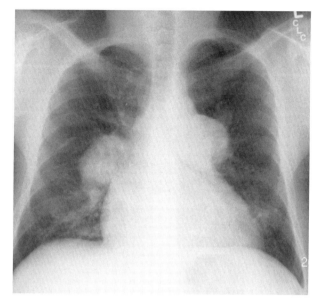

Figure 128A

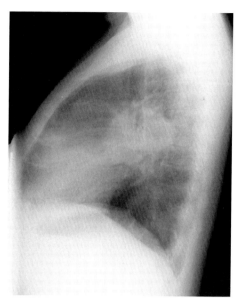

Figure 128B

Findings: PA and lateral radiographic views of the chest showed markedly enlarged hila bilaterally, with filling in of the AP window on the lateral chest film. The more peripheral pulmonary arteries rapidly tapered to a small caliber.

Diagnosis: Massive enlargement of the central pulmonary arteries from pulmonary hypertension with Eisenmenger's syndrome.

Discussion: This patient has severe pulmonary hypertension with massive central enlargement of the pulmonary arteries. He developed pulmonary hypertension from his VSD, with subsequent development of a right-to-left shunt, as well as severe hypoxemia, and presented for lung transplantation evaluation. He later declined all intervention except for supportive therapy.

His development of a right-to-left shunt from severe pulmonary hypertension is indicative of the development of Eisenmenger's complex. At this point the changes in pulmonary vascular resistance are irreversible, and because of the high pressures in the pulmonary vascular bed, the shunt across the VSD changes from a left-to-right to a right-to-left shunt.

Common causes of pulmonary hypertension include primary idiopathic pulmonary hypertension, chronic pulmonary thromboembolic disease, congenital heart disease with a left-to-right shunt (commonly VSD or atrial septal defect), and cor pulmonale.

CASE 129

History: The patient was a 62-year-old who underwent preoperative chest radiography prior to excision of a pelvic mass.

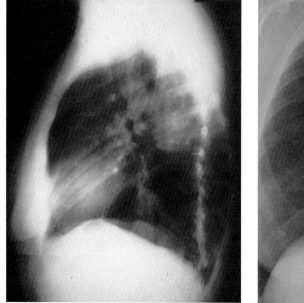

Figure 129A

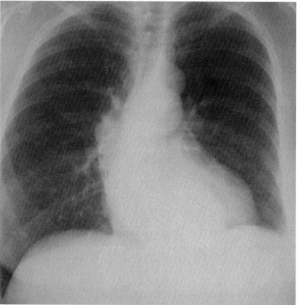

Figure 129B

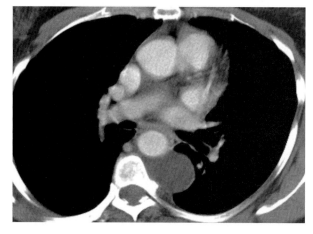

Figure 129C

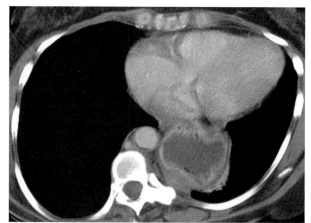

Figure 129D

Findings: PA and lateral chest radiographs demonstrated a soft tissue density in the posterior mediastinum, which measured approximately 4 cm in diameter. This was a rounded, smooth configuration and overlay the spine on the lateral view. CT was obtained for further characterization and showed a diffuse, low-attenuation mass without internal enhancement or calcifications. The mass was adjacent to the vertebral body in the left paraspinal location in the posterior mediastinum (*C*). A large hiatal hernia was also present (*D*).

Diagnosis: Bronchogenic cyst.

Discussion: Many paravertebral processes can be cystic in appearance. Abscess, metastases, and hematoma are probably the most commonly encountered entities. Other cystic masses in the posterior mediastinum include foregut duplication cysts, meningoceles, and meningomyeloceles. Occasionally, neurogenic neoplasms such as schwannoma or neurofibromas can have a cystic appearance. True cysts within the posterior mediastinum most likely are esophageal duplication cysts, neuroenteric cysts, or bronchogenic cysts.

Bronchogenic cysts are a type of foregut cyst resulting from abnormal budding or branching of the tracheobronchial tree. While the most common site is within the lung parenchyma (lower lobes), they can also occur within the mediastinum (posterior and middle mediastinum most common). Most are located near the carina when they occur within the mediastinum, with the subcarinal region being a particularly prevalent location. Histologically, bronchogenic cysts are lined with respiratory epithelium. The characteristic histologic feature is the presence of cartilage within the wall of the cyst. When located within the mediastinum, these cysts rarely communicate with the tracheobronchial tree. On CT, the masses are well defined with uniform low attenuation on CT. Calcifications are usually not present. On MRI, the high water content of the cyst yields bright signal intensity on T2-weighted images.

CASE 130

History: The patients were a 45-year-old woman presenting for routine preoperative assessment for elective surgery (*A, B*, chest radiography and CT) and a 36-year-old woman presenting for a routine chest radiograph on which an abnormality was detected. MRI was subsequently performed for further evaluation (*C, D*).

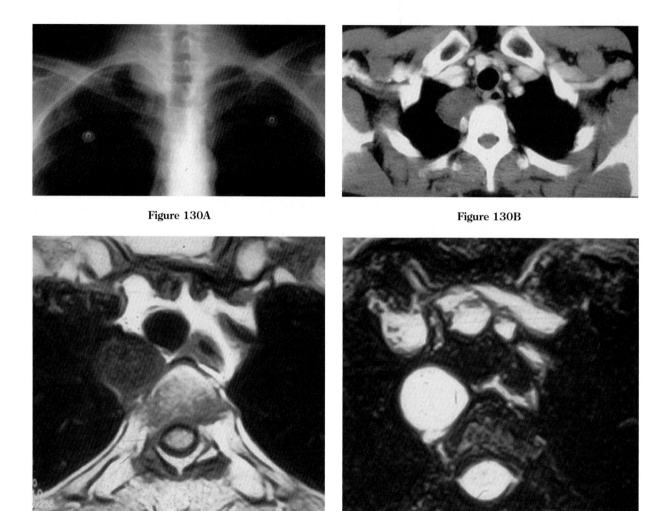

Figure 130A

Figure 130B

Figure 130C

Figure 130D

Findings: The cone-down view of a PA chest radiograph in the first patient demonstrated a rounded soft tissue density at the right lung apex medially in a paravertebral location. CT demonstrated a low-attenuation mass, which was uniformly of water density and contained no calcification or areas of enhancement. This was in a right paravertebral location adjacent to the esophagus and posterior to the trachea.

T1- and T2-weighted MRI images of the chest in the second patient demonstrated a smooth, rounded mass in the posterior mediastinum in a right paravertebral location. The mass was located posterior to the trachea and adjacent to the esophagus. The mass had uniformly low signal intensity on T1-weighted imaging and very high signal intensity, equal to that of the cerebrospinal fluid on T2-weighted imaging. No enhancement was seen with gadolinium-enhanced images.

Diagnosis: Esophageal duplication cyst.

Discussion: These two masses represent true cystic appearing masses within the posterior mediastinum. The most likely diagnosis would be an esophageal duplication cyst or a neuroenteric cyst. Neuroenteric cysts often have associated vertebral abnormalities and are connected to the meninges by a midline defect. They are often associated with the appearance of a hemivertebra.

Esophageal duplication cysts arise from the ventral foregut and the failure of embryologic development of the hollow structure. They are lined with gastrointestinal epithelium.

Cystic masses in the posterior mediastinum can be foregut cyst derivatives or false cysts from meningoceles, meningomyeloceles, or cystic-like entities such as other paravertebral processes. The masses depicted here have a truly cystic appearance, which is very bright on T2-weighted imaging. In terms of location and imaging characteristics, this case is a classic example of esophageal duplication cyst. They often occur high within the mediastinum near the apex of the lungs in the paravertebral location. MRI examination can be helpful in further evaluating suggested cystic masses of the mediastinum to evaluate their true cystic nature. Imaging is best done with long T2-weighted sequences as well as gadolinium-enhanced T1-weighted images. These lesions should have a thin and imperceptible wall with no evidence of enhancement with gadolinium.

CASE 131

History: The patient was a 22-year-old man with a long history of medical problems related to his present illness.

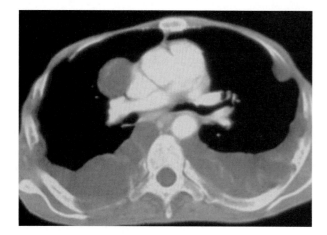

Figure 131A

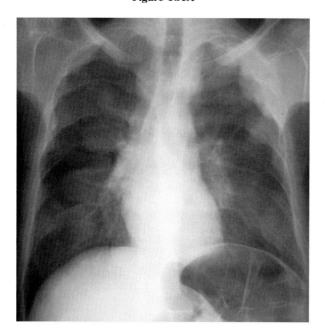

Figure 131B

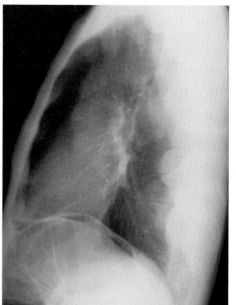

Figure 131C

Findings: PA and lateral chest radiographs showed multiple bilateral mediastinal masses that were located posteriorly on the lateral film. In addition, there were multiple large chest wall masses with associated erosive changes in the adjacent ribs. CT with contrast showed paraspinal masses with plexiform extension into the costovertebral spaces bilaterally with erosive rib changes evident. There also was a right middle mediastinal mass. The masses were low attenuation in nature with some internal enhancement evident.

Diagnosis: Neurofibromatosis (NF).

Discussion:

Neurofibroma

Neurofibromas can occur either as an isolated lesion or as part of NF. These tumors, like schwannomas, are peripheral nerve sheath spindle cell tumors. Their imaging appearance is similar to that of schwannomas, except that necrosis and hemorrhage is not as commonly encountered. Neurofibromas can be hemorrhagic, however, particularly when reaching a large size. The characteristic appearance of this soft tissue attenuation mass is that of a dumbbell-shaped tumor arising from the neuroforamen.

Sympathetic Ganglia Tumors

Sympathetic ganglia tumors range from benign ganglioneuromas to malignant ganglioneuroblastomas to highly malignant neuroblastomas. Once treated, neuroblastomas may mature and differentiate into ganglioneuromas. The posterior mediastinum is the second most involved site, with the adrenal glands being the most common site of origin. These are the most common neurogenic tumors encountered in children.

On imaging, these are large masses that often have associated bony erosions. Calcifications are also a frequent finding, occurring in both benign and malignant varieties.

Paraganglionic Tumors

Paraganglionic tumors, including pheochromocytomas and chemodectomas (paragangliomas), constitute the final category of neurogenic neoplasms. Chemodectomas arise from aortic bodies, which receive their sensory innervation from the 10th cranial nerve (vagus nerve).

These tumors are typically hypervascular, and thus may enhance brightly on CECT. They may be similarly bright on T2-weighted MRI. As with other neurogenic tumors, bony erosion is commonly seen. (Case courtesy of Dr. Jack Engelken.)

Key Imaging Features of Neurogenic Neoplasms

Large masses
Usually solid
Associated bony erosion
Calcifications common
Occasionally hemorrhagic

CASE 132

History: An 88-year-old man had a history of increasing shortness of breath and respiratory stridor over several preceding years, as well as increasing difficulty in swallowing.

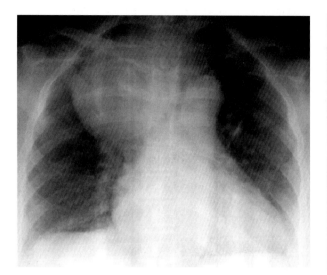

Figure 132A

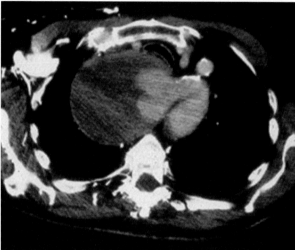

Figure 132B

Findings: The PA radiographic view of the chest showed a large right paratracheal mass that compressed and displaced the trachea to the left. A single image from contrast-enhanced CT of the chest showed the large retrotracheal masslike structure in continuity with the aortic arch, with some vascular enhancement within it. This structure had a significant mass effect upon the trachea, which was pushed anteriorly and flattened, and the esophagus, which was not well seen, but was located immediately posterior to the trachea and anterior to the masslike structure.

Diagnosis: Large aneurysm of an aberrant right subclavian artery.

Discussion: Aneurysms can have a cystic appearance on imaging. When encountered within the middle or posterior mediastinum, they most commonly arise from the aorta, although aneurysms of the great vessels, pulmonary arteries, and heart are also found within the mediastinum. These aneurysms are usually distinguishable as arising from one of the vascular structures mentioned above, especially on CECT, when contrast can be seen within nonthrombosed aneurysms. However, the recognition of thrombosed saccular aneurysms can be a diagnostic challenge on occasion, because they can appear as rounded masses adjacent to vascular structures, without obvious flow-related enhancement. In these cases, multiplanar imaging with MRI or three-dimensional reconstructions can aid in distinction of these masses as vascular in origin.

CASE 133

History: A 43-year-old man presented with a history of sharp chest and upper back pain of several days' duration. An abnormal chest radiograph in the emergency room led to further evaluation with CT.

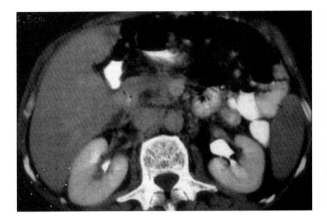

Figure 133A

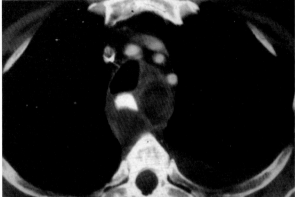

Figure 133B

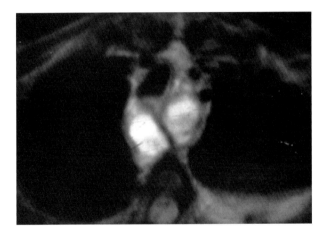

Figure 133C

Findings: CT of the chest with contrast showed several low-attenuation masslike densities in the posterior and middle mediastinum (*B*). These areas showed no real enhancement with contrast. MRI was subsequently obtained for further characterization. T2-weighted MRI showed the lesions to be of very high signal intensity (*C*). CT of the upper abdomen included on the chest CT showed enlargement of the pancreatic head with some peripancreatic stranding (*D*).

Diagnosis: Pancreatitis with pseudocyst involving the mediastinum.

Discussion: Many paravertebral processes can be cystic in appearance. Abscess, metastases, and hematoma are probably the most commonly encountered entities, however. Paravertebral abscesses may arise as a result of extension of infection from the adjacent vertebral bodies, meninges, mediastinum, or pleural space. Attenuation is near water density or of higher attenuation when the abscess contains more proteinaceous fluid or debris.

Hematomas are also of variable attenuation on CT (and variable signal intensity on MRI), depending on the age of the hematoma and the stage of the blood products contained within the hematoma. Associated vertebral or rib fractures are a common finding in the setting of trauma. Vascular injuries also may be a causative agent. Other entities that can appear as cystlike masses include hiatal or paraesophageal hernias and pancreatic pseudocysts.

Pseudocysts can occasionally extend above the diaphragm to involve the mediastinum, although this is a relatively rare occurrence. When they do, the inflammatory change often extends through the esophageal or aortic hiatus; thus, the posterior mediastinum is most commonly affected. A left-sided or bilateral pleural effusion is often seen in addition, although this is also commonly seen when pancreatitis is present that is confined to the abdomen and does not involve the mediastinum.

CASE 134

History: The patient was a 36-year-old woman with a history of a known congenital abnormality that had required multiple surgeries.

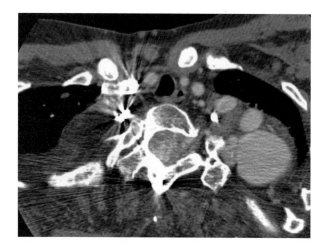

Figure 134A

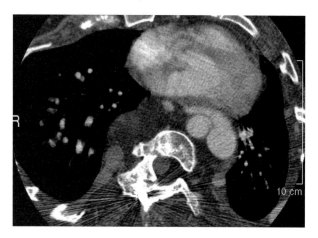

Figure 134B

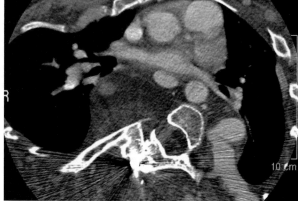

Figure 134C

Findings: Images from contrast-enhanced CT of the chest showed a markedly dilated hemiazygous vein with other enlarged paraspinal and chest wall collateral vessels in the left hemithorax. Scoliotic changes were present in the thoracic spine with enlargement of the spinal canal and a large enhancing mass within the spinal canal (*A*).

Diagnosis: Enlarged hemiazygous vein in a patient with Klippel-Trenaunay-Weber syndrome (KTWS) with numerous arteriovenous malformations of the thorax.

Discussion: This patient has KTWS, in which she produces large soft tissue hemangiomas. These have gradually (over many years) encroached on her thoracolumbar spine, producing a severe myelopathy. She has had numerous admissions for percutaneous embolization of these masses.

Klippel-Trenaunay syndrome is characterized by a triad of bony and soft tissue hypertrophy involving an extremity, port-wine stain, and varicose veins. The leg is the most common site of involvement, followed by the arms, trunk, and rarely the head and neck. Usually only a single extremity is involved. Discrepancies in limb length of up to 12 cm have been reported in the literature.

Most cases are sporadic, although a few cases in the literature report an autosomal-dominant pattern of inheritance.

Visceral organs such as the pleura, liver, spleen, urinary bladder, and gastrointestinal tract also may be involved. This patient had involvement of her spleen in addition to the spine and chest wall.

CASE 135

History: A 27-year-old Hispanic woman had a previous history of a primitive neuroectodermal tumor with positive Ewing's sarcoma markers involving her left abdominal wall. She originally presented with a rapidly enlarging mass located on her left lower abdominal wall, which had grown from the size of a marble to 6 to 7 cm over the course of several months. This was surgically excised. She had recent onset of increasing right chest pain, and a chest radiograph and CT were subsequently performed.

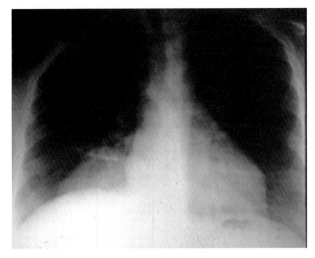

Figure 135A

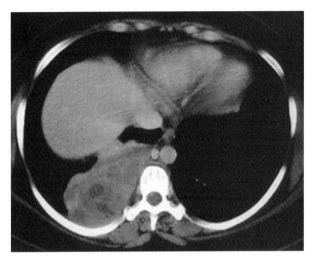

Figure 135B

Findings: A PA radiographic view of the chest showed a large mass behind the cardiac silhouette on the right. The mass was distinct from the right heart border and thus can be placed in all likelihood posteriorly. CT demonstrated a large enhancing right posterior mediastinal mass extending laterally and posteriorly in the costophrenic sulcus posteriorly.

Diagnosis: Metastases to the right paravertebral space from primitive neuroectodermal tumor (PNET).

Discussion: PNET, also known as neuroepithelioma, is included in the Ewing family of tumors, which also includes Ewing's tumor of bone, extraosseus Ewing's, and Askin's tumor (PNET of the chest wall). These tumors have an unfavorable prognosis in general, with the most favorable sites of involvement being the distal extremities and central location, such as the skull, clavicle or vertebrae, and ribs. Lesions involving the proximal extremities, especially the pelvis, have a much worse prognosis. Surgical resectability plays an important role in prognosis, but the most effective treatment is resection followed by adjuvant radiation and chemotherapy.

Metastases are included in the differential diagnosis of patients with a paravertebral mass and a known primary lesion. They can have a cystic or solid appearance dependent on the nature of the primary lesion and the degree of central necrosis. Metastases can be from any primary lesion, with common primary lesions including bronchogenic carcinoma, neuroectodermal tumors, and neurogenic neoplasms.

CASE 136

History: A 6-year-old boy had undergone multiple follow-up examinations for his chronic underlying disease. He was developmentally normal but had a large mass on his anterior chest wall and had undergone numerous spinal surgeries for kyphoscoliosis.

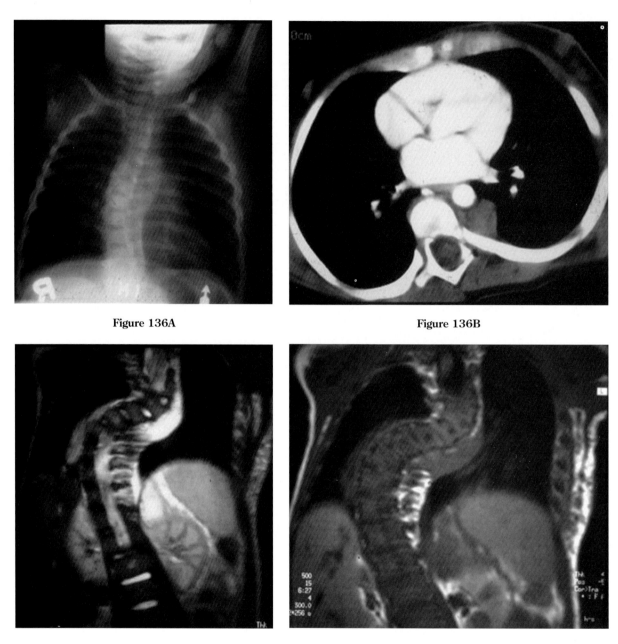

Figure 136A

Figure 136B

Figure 136C

Figure 136D

Findings: A PA radiographic view of the chest was obtained at approximately 15 months of age and showed scoliosis of the thoracic spine with extensive paravertebral masses evident bilaterally. CT of the chest obtained years later shows a left paravertebral mass that was of uniform low attenuation. Coronal T2-weighted (*C*) and T1-weighted (TR 500, TE 35) MRI (*D*) was performed as a follow-up examination and showed bilateral paravertebral masses that were very bright on T2-weighed imaging and dark on T1-weighted imaging. There was plexiform extension along the spine with worsening kyphoscoliosis.

Diagnosis: Neurofibromatosis type 1.

Discussion: NF has been classified into two distinct types: NF1 and NF2.

Neurofibromatosis type 1 occurs with an incidence of 1 in 4,000 births and is characterized by multiple cafe-au-lait spots and cutaneous neurofibromas. There is often associated deformation of bones and kyphoscoliosis of the spine. Other names for NF1 include von Recklinghausen NF and peripheral NF.

Neurofibromatosis type 2 is much rarer, occurring with an incidence of 1 in 40,000 births. NF2 is characterized by multiple tumors on the cranial and spinal nerves, most commonly acoustic neuromas involving the eighth cranial nerve, and by other lesions of the brain and spinal cord, including meningiomas and schwannomas. Hearing loss beginning in the teens or early twenties is generally the first symptom.

Both forms of NF are autosomal-dominant genetic disorders that may be inherited from a parent who has NF or may be the result of a spontaneous mutation. NF1 is associated with an abnormal locus on chromosome 17 (17q11), and NF2 is associated with an abnormal locus on chromosome 22. This child's mother had NF1 as well.

CASE 137

History: A 25-year-old white woman was in her normal state of good health when she experienced chest fullness and shortness of breath with anxiety. She presented to the emergency room, and chest radiography was performed.

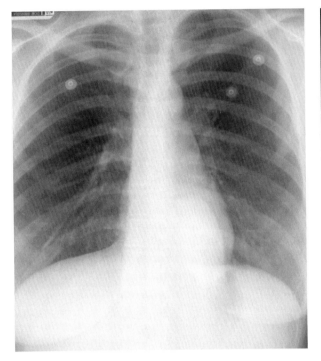

Figure 137A

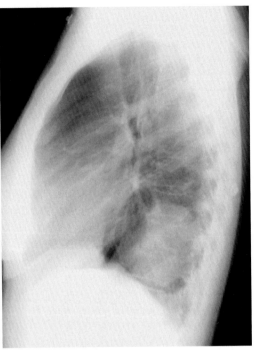

Figure 137B

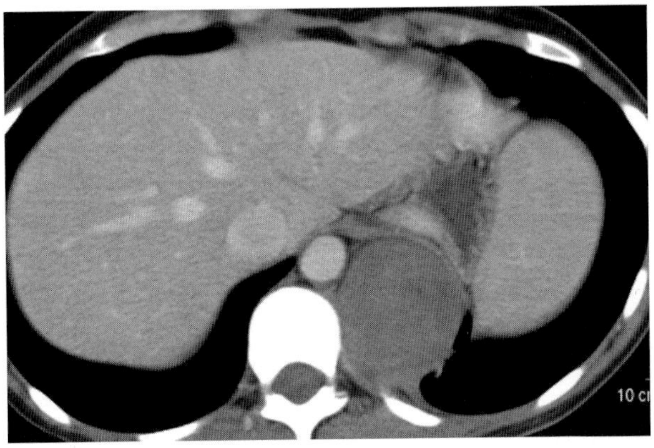

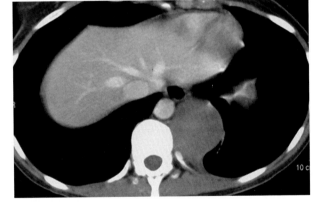

Figure 137C

Figure 137D

Findings: PA and lateral chest radiographs showed a large left posterior mediastinal mass that was distinct from the cardiac silhouette. Contrast-enhanced CT showed an enhancing left paraspinal mass with retrocrural extension. The mass was well circumscribed and soft tissue in attenuation.

Diagnosis: Schwannoma.

Discussion: Schwannoma, like neurofibroma, is a benign neoplasm originating from the peripheral nerve sheath and constitutes the most common neurogenic tumor of the posterior mediastinum. In the thorax, schwannomas may involve the intercostal, vagal, or phrenic nerves. These tumors, composed of spindle cells, are smooth and encapsulated and eccentrically located, with respect to the nerve of origin. They often contain areas of hemorrhage and necrosis.

Malignant schwannomas are rare (2% of all cases), but they are slightly more common in patients with underlying NF1 and are characterized by rapid growth and local invasion, rather than distant metastases.

Imaging shows a sharply demarcated paravertebral mass, which often has associated bony erosive changes (spinal canal or neuroforamen). Attenuation may be water density or less, secondary to the cystic areas of necrosis and hemorrhage. In addition, calcifications are occasionally seen (approximately 10%) within the mass. On MRI, schwannomas have low to intermediate signal on T1 images, with enhancement following gadolinium administration, and intermediate to high signal on T2 images.

Key Imaging Findings of Schwannoma

Smooth, round mass
Necrosis and hemorrhage
Occasional calcifications
Low attenuation
Associated bony erosions

SUGGESTED READING

Alexander F. Neuroblastoma. *Urol Clin North Am* 2000;27:383–392, vii.

Ambros IM, Ambros PF, Strehl S, et al. MIC2 is a specific marker for Ewing sarcoma and peripheral primitive neuroectodermal tumors. *Cancer* 1991;67:1886–1893.

Arenas-Jimenez J, Alonso-Charterina S, Sanchez-Paya J, et al. Evaluation of CT findings for diagnosis of pleural effusions. *Eur Radiol* 2000;10:681–690.

Cangemi V, Volpino P, Gualdi G, et al. Pericardial cysts of the mediastinum. *J Cardiovasc Surg (Torino)* 1999;40:909–913.

Ching AS, Chan PN, Cheung H, et al. CT and DSA appearances of a ruptured congenital arteriovenous malformation of the posterior mediastinal aorta. *Br J Radiol* 2000;73:1320–1322.

Divisi D, Battaglia C, Crisci R, et al. Diagnostic and therapeutic approaches for masses in the posterior mediastinum. *Acta Biomed Ateneo Parmense* 1998;69:123–128.

Erasmus JJ, McAdams HP, Donnelly LF, et al. MR imaging of mediastinal masses. *Magn Reson Imaging Clin North Am* 2000;8:59–89.

Frizzera G, Moran EM, Rappaport H. Angioimmunoblastic lymphadenopathy with dysproteinaemia. *Lancet* 1976;1:1070–1073.

Frizzera G, Moran EM, Rappaport H. Angioimmunoblastic lymphadenopathy. Diagnosis and clinical course. *Am J Med* 1975;59:803–818.

Garrett HE Jr., Roper CL. Surgical intervention in histoplasmosis. *Ann Thorac Surg* 1986;42:711.

Hoeffel C, Floquet J, Regent D, et al. Periesophageal mediastinal fibromatosis. *Abdom Imaging* 2000;25:235–238.

Jung KJ, Lee KS, Han J, et al. Malignant thymic epithelial tumors: CT-pathologic correlation. *AJR Am J Roentgenol* 2001;176:433–439.

Ketai L, Brandt MM, Schermer C. Nonaortic mediastinal injuries from blunt chest trauma. *J Thorac Imaging* 2000;15:120–127.

Kim Y, Lee KS, Yoo JH, et al. Middle mediastinal lesions: imaging findings and pathologic correlation. *Eur J Radiol* 2000;35:30–38.

Kirchner S, Hernanz-Schulman M, Stein SM, et al. Imaging of pediatric mediastinal histoplasmosis. *Radiographics* 1991;11:365–381.

Kirchner SG, Heller RM, Smith CW. Pancreatic pseudocyst of the mediastinum. *Radiology* 1977;123:37–42.

Kono T, Kohno A, Kuwashima S, et al. CT findings of descending necrotising mediastinitis via the carotid space. *Pediatr Radiol* 2001;31:84–86.

Kwak HS, Lee JM. CT findings of extramedullary hematopoiesis in the thorax, liver and kidneys, in a patient with idiopathic myelofibrosis. *J Korean Med Sci* 2000;15:460–462.

Landay M, Rollins N. Mediastinal histoplasmosis granuloma: evaluation with CT. *Radiology* 1989;172:657.

Lee DK, Im JG, Lee KS, et al. B-cell lymphoma of bronchus-associated lymphoid tissue (BALT): CT features in 10 patients. *J Comput Assist Tomogr* 2000;24:30–34.

Lee JY, Lee KS, Jung KJ, et al. Pulmonary tuberculosis: CT and pathologic correlation. *J Comput Assist Tomogr* 2000;24:691–698.

Leissa B. Histoplasmosis. In: Feigin, Cherry, eds. *Textbook of pediatric infectious diseases*. Philadelphia: WB Saunders, 1992.

Loyd J, Tillman BF, Atkinson JB, et al. Mediastinal fibrosis complicating histoplasmosis. *Medicine (Baltimore)* 1988;67:295–310.

Loyer E, Fuller L, Libshitz HI, et al. Radiographic appearance of the chest following therapy for Hodgkin disease. *Eur J Radiol* 2000;35:136–148.

Mathew P, Roberts JA, Zwischenberger J, Haque AK. Mediastinal atypical carcinoid and neurofibromatosis type 1. *Arch Pathol Lab Med* 2000;124:319–321.

Myers JL, Gomes MN. Management of aberrant subclavian artery aneurysms. *J Cardiovasc Surg (Torino)* 2000;41:607–612.

Ngom A, Dumont P, Diot P, et al. Benign mediastinal lymphadenopathy in congestive heart failure. *Chest* 2001;119:653–656.

Protopapas Z, Westcott JL. Transthoracic hilar and mediastinal biopsy. *Radiol Clin North Am* 2000;38:281–291.

Salo JA, Savola JK, Toikkanen VJ, et al. Successful treatment of mediastinal gas gangrene due to esophageal perforation. *Ann Thorac Surg* 2000;70:2143–2145.

Schulman H, Newman-Heinman N, Kurtzbart E, et al. Thoracoabdominal peripheral primitive neuroectodermal tumors in childhood: radiological features. *Eur Radiol* 2000;10:1649–1652.

Strollo DC, Rosado-de-Christenson ML, Jett JR. Primary mediastinal tumors. Part II: Tumors of the middle and posterior mediastinum. *Chest* 1997;112:1344–1357.

Sugio KK, Ondo KK, Yamaguchi MM, et al. Thymoma arising in a thymic cyst. *Ann Thorac Cardiovasc Surg* 2000;6:329–331.

Tanaka A, Takeda R, Utsunomiya H, et al. Severe complications of mediastinal pancreatic pseudocyst: report of esophagobronchial fistula and hemothorax. *J Hepatobiliary Pancreat Surg* 2000;7:86–91.

Thompson BH, Stanford W. MR imaging of pulmonary and mediastinal malignancies. *Magn Reson Imaging Clin North Am* 2000;8:729–739.

Topcu S, Alper A, Gulhan E, et al. Neurogenic tumours of the mediastinum: a report of 60 cases. *Can Respir J* 2000;7:261–265.

Van Putten JW, Schlosser NJ, Vujaskovic Z, et al. Superior vena cava obstruction caused by radiation induced venous fibrosis. *Thorax* 2000;55:245–246.

Weber AL, Randolph G, Aksoy FG. The thyroid and parathyroid glands. CT and MR imaging and correlation with pathology and clinical findings. *Radiol Clin North Am* 2000;38:1105–1129.

Weiland K, Conley J. A primary germ cell tumor of the anterior mediastinum: a case report and discussion. *S D J Med* 2000;53:441–444.

Wittich GR, Karnel F, Schurawitzki H, et al. Percutaneous drainage of mediastinal pseudocysts. *Radiology* 1988;167:51–53.

CHAPTER 8

THE PLEURA

MICHAEL J. JURGENS
PATRICIA J. MERGO

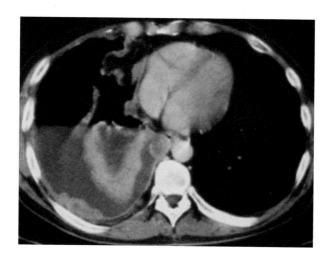

CASE 138

History: A 48-year-old man had sustained a gunshot wound to the left chest. He was discharged home after the chest tube had been removed, but returned 2 weeks later with fevers, chills, and left pleuritic chest pain.

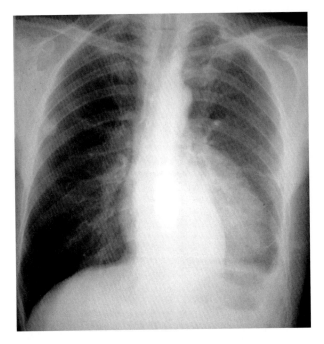

Figure 138A

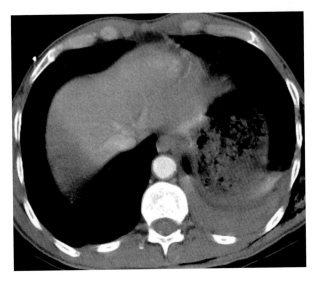

Figure 138B

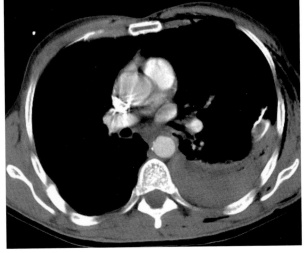

Figure 138C

Findings: Chest radiography at the 2-week follow-up examination showed a large rounded retrocardiac density that was distinct from the heart border and could be seen through the hemidiaphragm on the left. Two images from CT of the chest with contrast showed a left pleural fluid collection with high-density material within it consistent with blood or proteinaceous material. A left-sided chest tube was also in place.

Differential Diagnosis: Traumatic pleural effusion secondary to pleural injury, intercostal artery tear, aortic injury, and esophageal rupture should be considered.

Diagnosis: Pleural hematoma, with subsequent development of an empyema.

Discussion: Pleural effusions are often seen following penetrating or nonpenetrating trauma. The majority of pleural collections are due to hemorrhage. Only 10% of cases require surgery. Indications for surgical intervention include a bleeding rate greater than 200 mL/h or effusion greater than 1 L at presentation. Brisk bleeds are usually due to laceration of intercostal arteries or internal mammary or large mediastinal vessels. Other causes of traumatic hemothorax include laceration of the parietal or visceral pleura by fractured ribs or closed chest trauma without rib fracture. Traumatic rupture of the aorta causes a left-sided effusion. Esophageal rupture also causes a left-sided effusion with diagnostic ingested material in the pleural fluid.

Other traumatic causes of pleural effusion include trauma to the thoracic duct or diaphragm. Central venous catheters can perforate a vessel at the time of insertion or by gradual erosion through the vessel wall by a catheter tip.

On erect chest radiography, pleural effusions have a well-defined superior border, convex downward and blunting of the costophrenic angle. On supine films, the effusion layers in the dependent pleural space causing opacification of the entire lung. Subpulmonic effusions cause the usual mid-peak of the diaphragm to be displaced laterally.

CASE 139

History: A 69-year-old white man with esophageal squamous cell carcinoma had undergone esophagectomy with gastropharyngoscopy 4 months earlier. He presented to the emergency room with shortness of breath.

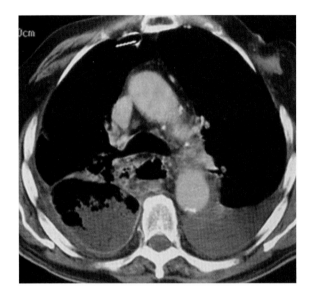 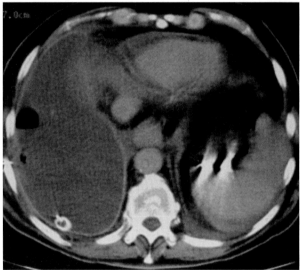

| Figure 139A | Figure 139B |

Findings: CT of the chest with contrast showed a large right pleural fluid collection with an air-fluid level present within the collection. Enhancement of the pleura on the right indicated an associated pleural inflammatory reaction. Subpleural fat deposition was noted bilaterally.

Differential Diagnosis: Empyema. Thoracentesis showed 200 red blood cells/mL, 375 white blood cells/mL, 99% polymorphonuclear cells, 1% monocytes, a glucose level of 4 mg/dL, and an LDH level of 1,175 U/L and a pH of 6.86. No organisms were seen on Gram stain. A chest tube was placed, and the patient's respiratory status improved. Eventually, the tube was converted to an empyema tube and the patient went home.

Diagnosis: Empyema.

Discussion: Infectious pleural effusions are exudative. The most common causes are bacterial (usually anaerobic), parapneumonic, tuberculous, fungal, and parasitic. An empyema is an exudative effusion with pus in the pleural cavity. Criteria for diagnosis include gross pus, organisms on stain or culture, white blood cell count greater than 5×10^9 cells/L, a pH less than 7.2, an LDH of greater than 1,000 U/L, and a glucose level of less than 40 mg/dL. Empyemas are usually caused by bacterial pneumonia or abscess but may follow thoracic surgery or trauma. If diagnostic aspiration shows infection by Gram stain or culture, then drainage is indicated.

There are three stages of empyema. Stage I is the *exudative stage* (sterile exudate) with elevated PMNs, a pH of greater than 7.20, and a glucose level of less than 40 mg/dL. Stage II is the *fibropurulent stage* and is divided into early and late stages. The early stage has increasing WBCs, pH of 7.0 to 7.2, and a glucose level of greater than 40 mg/dL. The late stage has gross pus, a pH of less than 7.0, and a glucose level of less than 40 mg/dL. Stage III is the *organization stage*, with fibroblast infiltration forming a pleural peel. This stage can occur as early as 7 days after the initial event if untreated and may require surgical decortication. Otherwise, pleural fibrosis may occur.

Clinical manifestations of pleural effusion include pleural pain described as a dull ache that can usually be localized. Dyspnea is also common. For severe dyspnea, immediate thoracentesis may be needed for symptomatic relief.

Radiographic findings are similar to those of a classic pleural effusion. When the effusion is loculated, no shift in positioning of the fluid is evident on decubitus imaging. The definitive diagnosis between sterile pleural effusion and empyema is made by thoracentesis, but certain CT findings are suggestive of empyema. On CT there is a split pleura sign. The pleura enhances with contrast and splits around the empyema. The extrapleural fat also is thickened, as seen in this case. Empyemas have a lenticular shape, form obtuse angles with the chest wall, and compress the surrounding lung, causing surrounding vessels to drape around it. In contradistinction, a lung abscess is round, forms an acute angle with the chest wall, and vessels of the lung end abruptly at the margins of the abscess.

CASE 140

History: A 51-year-old white man presented with back pain, dyspnea, weight loss, and night sweats. Chest radiography showed a right hydropneumothorax, and CT of the chest was subsequently performed for further evaluation.

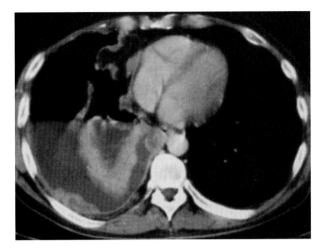

Figure 140A

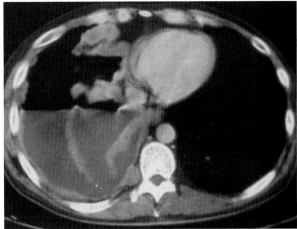

Figure 140B

Findings: CT showed a right hydropneumothorax with irregular, nodular thickening and enhancement of both the visceral and parietal pleura, with atelectasis of the right lower lobe.

Differential Diagnosis: Diffuse malignant mesothelioma of the pleura. On further questioning, the patient reported that he was exposed to asbestos while working in shipyards in the navy. Pleural biopsy confirmed the diagnosis of mesothelioma.

Diagnosis: Diffuse malignant mesothelioma of the pleura.

Discussion: Diffuse malignant mesothelioma of the pleura is becoming increasingly recognized, affecting 7 to 13 persons per million. Eighty percent of all patients have a history of occupational exposure to asbestos, but there is no relation to the duration or degree of exposure. Additionally, there is a latent period between exposure and clinical signs that usually exceeds 20 years and may extend up to 40 years.

Clinically, these patients present with vague chest or shoulder ache or true pleuritic pain. This can develop into shortness of breath, weight loss, and cough with the progression of disease. Many patients (90% in one study) have electrocardiographic abnormalities such as arrhythmias and conduction abnormalities. Patients often have extension through the chest wall and diaphragm with peritoneal mesothelioma. But symptomatology is usually confined to chest disease.

Confirming the diagnosis is difficult with cytology from pleural fluid because mesothelioma can be confused with metastatic adenocarcinoma, and distinction from reactive mesothelial inflammatory cells may be difficult. Therefore, a core pleural biopsy is usually needed to establish the diagnosis. There are three histologic types: epithelial, mesenchymal, and biphasic (mixed).

The prognosis for mesothelioma is extremely poor. Most patients die within 1 year of the onset of symptoms. Surgical resection consisting of en bloc excision of lung, parietal pleura, pericardium, diaphragm, and attached tumor offers some benefit in selected patients, but operative mortality from this surgery is not uncommon.

Radiographic findings usually include diffuse, irregular, nodular opacities encasing the periphery of the entire lung. A pleural effusion may or may not be present, but when present, the effusion usually will not cause a shift of mediastinal structures.

Fifty percent of patients have associated pleural plaques. CT and MRI can better demonstrate these features compared with plain film radiography and give a better impression of the full extent of disease for treatment planning.

CASE 141

History: A 64-year-old white woman with a recent diagnosis of squamous cell carcinoma of the lung had undergone several cycles of chemotherapy and presented with fever and cough.

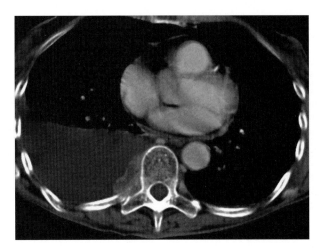

Figure 141

Findings: CT of the chest with contrast showed nodular, enhancing, irregular pleural thickening in the posterior right hemithorax, immediately adjacent to the spine. There was also a large right-sided pleural effusion.

Differential Diagnosis: Metastatic lung cancer. On follow-up CT scans, the patient's lung cancer had also spread to her thoracic spine.

Diagnosis: Metastatic lung cancer to the pleura.

Discussion: Clinically, patients with carcinoma of the pleura usually present with symptoms due to their large pleural effusion, including dyspnea on exertion, and cough. Because of the advanced state of their disease, these patients have substantial weight loss and appear chronically ill. Unfortunately, when bronchogenic carcinoma involves the pleura diffusely with a resultant pleural effusion, the tumor is considered unresectable. It is important to establish the cause of the effusion because 5% of these patients have an effusion from a different cause and should not be considered inoperable. The prognosis is extremely poor, with a survival time of only a few months from diagnosis of the malignant effusion.

Metastatic disease is the second leading cause of pleural effusion after congestive heart failure in patients over 50 years of age. In fact, 25% of all pleural effusions in older patients are malignant in origin. The effusion is usually caused by impaired lymphatic drainage, and there may be no direct pleural involvement with tumor. CT plays a role in differentiating benign from malignant pleural disease. There are four features that are highly specific for metastatic disease: circumferential pleural thickening, nodular pleural thickening, parietal pleural thickening of greater than 1 cm, and mediastinal pleural involvement.

CASE 142

History: An 83-year-old man presented with a 6-week history of a cough.

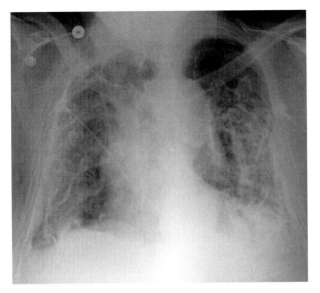

Figure 142A

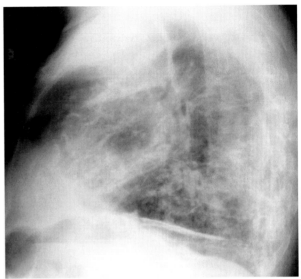

Figure 142B

Findings: Chest radiography showed diffuse bilateral pleural plaques, many of which were calcified, and irregular bilateral pleural thickening.

Differential Diagnosis: Asbestos-related pleural disease. The patient reported a 6-year exposure to asbestos from 1948 to 1954.

Diagnosis: Asbestos-related pleural disease.

Discussion: Asbestos is composed of a group of minerals that are fibrous and resistant to high temperatures and chemical insults. They are divided into two major groups: curved fibers and straight fibers. There are three main sources of exposure: (a) primary exposure from asbestos mining and its processing in a mill; (b) secondary exposure from its use in industrial and commercial products such as construction, the automotive industry, and shipbuilding; and (c) airborne exposure of persons who are not in asbestos-related occupations.

Clinically, there is a latent period of 20 to 40 years between exposure and disease. The majority of patients are asymptomatic. They may have pleural pain associated with a pleural effusion. In the late stages, they may develop shortness of breath from interstitial fibrosis. On examination, these patients have crackles in the lung bases. This finding, associated with a history of asbestos exposure, is sufficient to make a diagnosis of asbestosis. A pulmonary function test will show a restrictive pattern.

Asbestos-related pleural disease has several manifestations. Pleural plaques may be smooth or nodular and are usually thin. They are on the parietal pleura overlying the ribs and the domes of the diaphragm, sparing the apices, costophrenic angles, and anterior chest wall. They are usually multiple, bilateral, and involve posterolateral ribs 7 to 10 and lateral ribs 6 to 9. They are often difficult to distinguish on radiography from fat and muscle shadows. These patients also can have focal or diffuse pleural fibrosis. This is seen on radiography as diffuse pleural thickening or thickening of interlobular fissures. Pleural effusion is often the only finding seen in the first 20 years following asbestos exposure.

Pulmonary asbestosis is the term reserved for diffuse parenchymal interstitial fibrosis, most commonly in the subpleural regions of the lower lobes. The lung changes occur in three stages. First, a fine reticulation pattern with associated ground-glass appearance occurs, predominantly in the lower lung zones. Then, the reticular pattern becomes more prominent. In the late stage, the reticulation is severe and may involve all lung zones. CT shows similar findings and may show round atelectasis with a classic "comet tail."

CASE 143

History: A 30-year-old woman presented with abdominal pain. Her past medical history was significant only for splenectomy following a motor vehicle accident 14 years earlier. Chest radiography from an obstructive series showed a pleural-based mass, prompting a CT scan of the chest.

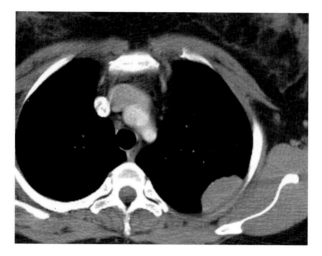

Figure 143A

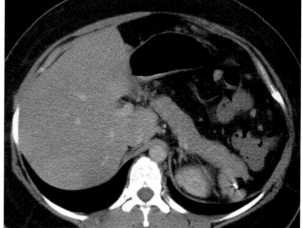

Figure 143B

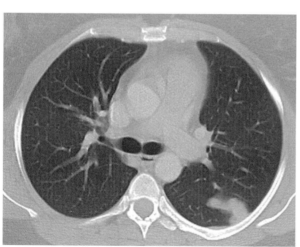

Figure 143C

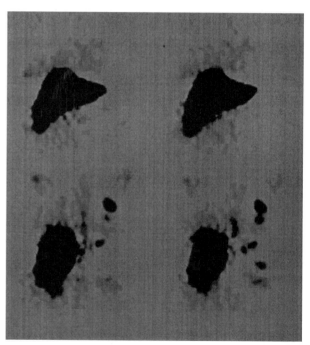

Figure 143D

Findings: There were three large soft tissue masses at the periphery of the left lung. CT of the chest with contrast showed one of the pleural masses (*A*), which had a smooth, lobulated contour. A CT image in the lung windows showed a second mass located within the fissure on the left (*C*). Axial CT of the upper abdomen showed that the patient had undergone splenectomy (*B*).

Differential Diagnosis: Pleural metastases or intrathoracic splenosis should be considered. A liver-spleen scan showed radiotracer uptake in three masses in the posterior left chest and in two foci in the left upper quadrant, consistent with regenerating splenic tissue.

Diagnosis: Thoracic splenosis.

Discussion: Thoracic splenosis is a rare entity in which autotransplantation of splenic tissue occurs into the pleural cavity. Typically, following rupture of the spleen, fragments of splenic tissue seed the peritoneal cavity. If there is diaphragmatic injury at the time of the splenic rupture, splenic tissue can implant on the pleura. The reported cases have a time lapse between the initial injury and the discovery of the thoracic mass of 9 to 32 years.

Diagnosis used to be made with surgical resection. Currently, the diagnosis is made with nuclear medicine, using technetium 99m sulfur colloid, indium 111 platelets, or technetium 99m heat-damaged red blood cells. These scans will show an increased uptake at the same location as the pleural mass found on CT. Because nuclear medicine scans are not a typical study performed in the workup of chest masses, a high index of suspicion is needed. Absence of Howell-Jolly bodies, pitted erythrocytes, and siderocytes in asplenic patients suggest the presence of residual splenic tissue. If the masses are subpleural and scattered in the chest, and the patient has a history of thoracoabdominal trauma, thoracic splenosis should be considered.

There has been no reported morbidity or mortality with thoracic splenosis. Therefore, the current recommendations are against surgical resection. Instead, patients are monitored with yearly chest radiography to evaluate for growth or interval change in the splenosis. The astute physician will thus avoid for their patient a trip to the operating room.

CASE 144

History: A 46-year-old woman with a history of thymoma had undergone chemotherapy, resection, and radiation therapy. Prior CT scans had shown no progression of disease. The patient presented with back pain.

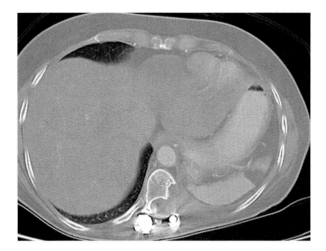

Figure 144A

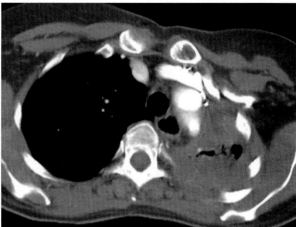

Figure 144B

Findings: Axial CT images of the chest with contrast showed soft tissue surrounding the aorta and destroying a lower thoracic vertebral body and pedicle, with expansion of the spinal canal. There was also a soft tissue mass at the apical portion of the left lung that had eroded through the chest wall.

Differential Diagnosis: Pleural metastases. Biopsy confirmed the diagnosis of malignant thymoma metastatic to the pleura and left chest wall.

Diagnosis: Thymoma metastases.

Discussion: Solid pleural metastases can occur from direct pleural seeding, usually from intrathoracic tumors. This is seen with bronchogenic carcinoma and malignant thymoma. Invasive thymoma also may involve the pleura by direct contiguous spread. Pleural seeding often is seen as a recurrence of disease following surgical resection and represents one of the most common sites of metastatic foci from invasive thymoma, because invasive thymoma has a known propensity for spread to the pleural space and pericardium. Therefore, careful follow-up with CT is recommended to determine the presence of recurrence. The CT findings include pleural seeding, which typically appears as small plaquelike areas of pleural thickening.

Pleural metastases are the most common pleural neoplasm (95% of cases). Findings of metastatic disease to the pleura usually include a large pleural effusion, but also may include pleural nodules or extensive pleural thickening. This can be difficult to differentiate from malignant mesothelioma. The most common primaries are bronchogenic carcinoma (35%), breast cancer (25%), lymphoma (10%), and ovarian or gastric cancer (<5% each), with 15% other and 10% unknown.

SUGGESTED READING

Arenas-Jimenez J, Alonso-Charterina S, Sanchez-Paya J, et al. Evaluation of CT findings for diagnosis of pleural effusions. *Eur Radiol* 2000; 10:681–690.

Baber CE, Hedlund LW, Oddson TA, et al. Differentiating empyemas and peripheral pulmonary abscesses: the value of computed tomography. *Radiology* 1980;135:755–758.

Gallardo X, Castaner E, Mata JM. Benign pleural diseases. *Eur J Radiol* 2000;34:87–97.

Knisely BL, Kuhlman JE. Radiographic and computed tomography (CT) imaging of complex pleural disease. *Crit Rev Diagn Imaging* 1997; 38:1–58.

Kuhlman JE, Singha NK. Complex disease of the pleural space: radiographic and CT evaluation. *Radiographics* 1997;17:63–79.

McLoud TC, Flower CD. Imaging the pleura: sonography, CT, and MR imaging. *AJR Am J Roentgenol* 1991;156:1145–1153.

Miller A. Asbestos-related bilateral diffuse pleural thickening: natural history of radiographic and lung function abnormalities. *Am J Respir Crit Care Med* 1996;154(part 1):1919–1920.

Mintzer RA, Gore RM, Vogelzang RL, et al. Rounded atelectasis and its association with asbestos-induced pleural disease. *Radiology* 1981; 139:567–570.

Muller NL. Imaging of the pleura. *Radiology* 1993;186 297–309.

Oksa P, Huuskonen MS, Jarvisalo J, et al. Follow-up of asbestosis patients and predictors for radiographic progression. *Int Arch Occup Environ Health* 1998;71:465–471.

Roucos S. Thoracic splenosis. *Thorac Cardiovasc Surg* 1990;99:361–363.

Sahn SA. Pleural diseases related to metastatic malignancies. *Eur Respir J* 1997;10:1648–1654.

Soysal O, Karaoglanoglu N, Demiracan S, et al. Pleurectomy/decortication for palliation in malignant pleural mesothelioma: results of surgery. *Eur J Cardiothorac Surg* 1997;11:210–213.

Tsunezuka Y, Sato H. Thoracic splenosis; from a thoracoscopic viewpoint. *Eur J Cardiothorac Surg* 1998;13:104–106.

Wilson RW, Gallateau-Salle F, Moran CA. Desmoid tumors of the pleura: a clinicopathologic mimic of localized fibrous tumor. *Mod Pathol* 1999;12:9–14.

Woodring JH. Pleural effusion is a cause of round atelectasis of the lung. *J Ky Med Assoc* 2000;98:527–532.

Youssem SA. Thoracic splenosis. *Ann Thorac Surg* 1987;44:411–412.

Zeren EH, Colby TV, Roggli VL. Silica-induced pleural disease: an unusual case mimicking malignant mesothelioma. *Chest* 1997;112: 1436–1438.

CHAPTER 9

ABNORMAL AIR COLLECTIONS

ALLISON E. TONKIN
PATRICIA J. MERGO

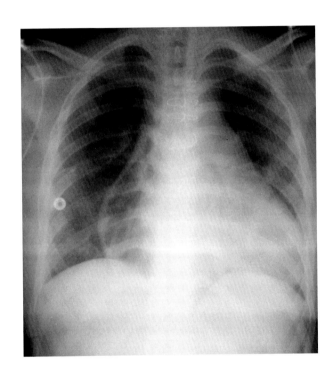

CASE 145

History: An 81-year-old man was admitted with 60% to 65% total body surface area burns and initially suffered an iatrogenic left pneumothorax at the time of a central venous catheter placement for intravenous fluid resuscitation. A left thoracostomy tube was placed with subsequent reexpansion of the left lung. The following chest film was obtained approximately 10 days after admission.

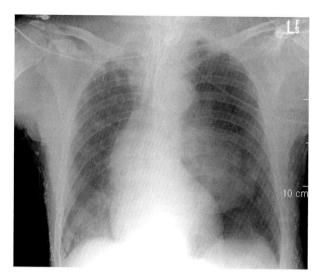

Figure 145

Findings: A frontal portable view of the chest demonstrated a large left pneumothorax with tension component evident by the rightward shift of mediastinal contents.

Diagnosis: Tension pneumothorax.

Discussion: Pneumothorax, the presence of air within the pleural space, is usually traumatic or iatrogenic in origin, but may occur spontaneously. A tension pneumothorax occurs when inspired air becomes trapped within the pleural space, presumably because of a bronchopleural check valve mechanism. Immediate recognition is essential because affected patients often rapidly become severely hypoxic and acidotic and may die.

There is extension of gas from the airspace of the pulmonary parenchyma into the interstitial tissues and then into the pleural space. In most patients there is usually an initial event of ascending increase in alveolar pressure, and gas extends peripherally in the interstitial tissues toward the visceral pleura and rupture into the pleural space to cause a pneumothorax. Underlying lung disease is a known contributory factor in the pathogenesis. Other contributing factors include the following: deep respiratory maneuvers (e.g., Valsalva), asthma (particularly in children), severe vomiting, positive end-expiratory pressure ventilation in patients with COPD or ARDS, closed chest trauma with shear forces, sudden drop in atmospheric pressure (rapid ascent of a scuba diver), or postoperatively following median sternotomy. Fracture or other disruption of the trachea or proximal main bronchi can result in pneumothorax. This may result from trauma, or it may occur following diagnostic instrumentation, such as bronchoscopic biopsy.

Pathologic specimens demonstrate an inflammatory reaction with a significant number of eosinophils brought on by the presence of air within the pleural space.

History: A 51-year-old Hispanic woman with a long history of asthma and bronchiectasis underwent bronchoscopy for biopsy of a 7-mm nodule in the right middle lobe. The patient tolerated the procedure well and was discharged home. Two to three hours later the patient presented to the emergency room with increasing shortness of breath, which was refractory to home nebulizer treatments. Physical examination revealed diffuse crepitus over the chest.

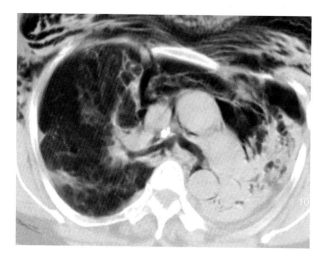

Figure 146A

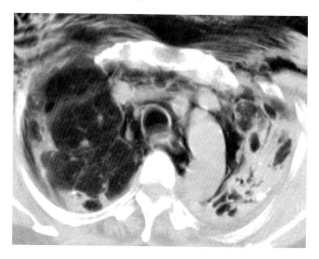

Figure 146B

Findings: Two axial images from a noncontrasted chest CT demonstrated pneumomediastinum and bilateral anterior pneumothoraces. Extensive subcutaneous emphysema in the soft tissues of the bilateral breasts, lateral soft tissues of the chest wall, and right posterior soft tissues was identified. Air outlines the mediastinal structures, including the ascending and descending aorta, trachea, and esophagus. The imaged lung parenchyma demonstrated extensive bronchiectasis with consolidation in the left upper lobe.

Diagnosis: Pneumomediastinum and bilateral pneumothoraces with associated extensive subcutaneous emphysema in a patient with significant bronchiectasis.

Discussion: Pneumomediastinum, or mediastinal emphysema, originates from one of five possible sites: lung, mediastinal airways, esophagus, neck, or abdominal cavity.

The chronic consolidative changes in the left lung were a result of long-standing inflammation from bronchiectasis and chronic relapsing infection. At bronchoscopy, biopsy samples were obtained in the region of a focal opacity, essentially creating a bronchopleural fistula. The extensive air collections described above are the direct result of this transient bronchopleural fistula. There is extension of gas from the airspace of the pulmonary parenchyma into the interstitial tissues, and then into the mediastinum. In most patients there is usually an initial event of ascending increase in alveolar pressure, often accompanied by airway narrowing, resulting in rupture of the alveoli adjacent to the airways or to the pulmonary arteries or veins.

Gas may extend proximally into the mediastinum to cause pneumomediastinum, or it may travel peripherally in the interstitial tissues toward the visceral pleura and rupture into the pleural space to cause a pneumothorax. Pneumothorax can often occur as a result of direct rupture of the mediastinum if there is sufficient gas accumulation. Mediastinal gas often tracks into the neck and subcutaneous tissues. It may extend into the retroperitoneum, and rarely, into the peritoneal space or spinal canal.

Contributing factors leading to pneumomediastinum are the same as those listed previously for pneumothorax. Fracture or other disruption of the trachea or proximal main bronchi can result in pneumomediastinum. This may result from trauma or it may occur following diagnostic instrumentation such as bronchoscopic biopsy.

Pathologic specimens demonstrate an inflammatory reaction with a significant number of eosinophils brought on by the presence of air within the mediastinum. This appearance is similar to that noted in the pleura in patients with pneumothorax.

Clinical manifestations of pneumomediastinum include subcutaneous emphysema and a history of abrupt onset of retrosternal pain radiating to the shoulders and arms. This is usually preceded by an event of excessive increase in intrathoracic pressure such as severe coughing, sneezing, or vomiting. Physical examination may demonstrate the presence of crepitus within the subcutaneous tissues in the neck. The Hamman sign on physical examination is the crunching or clicking noise synchronous with the heartbeat noted in approximately 50% of cases. This is best identified with the patient in the left lateral decubitus position. It should be noted that although this finding is characteristic of pneumomediastinum, it is not pathognomonic. If the air trapped within the mediastinum is not allowed to escape freely into the soft tissues, patients may present with engorged neck veins, a rapid thready pulse, and hypotension.

CASE 147

History: A 21-year-old woman had a history of aortic insufficiency after having recently undergone homograft replacement of the aortic valve.

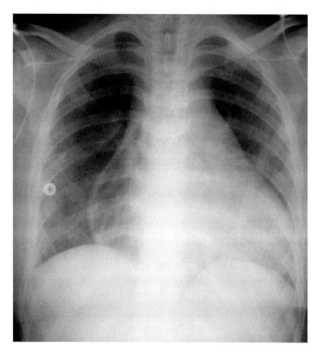

Figure 147

Findings: A single portable frontal view of the chest demonstrated postoperative changes of median sternotomy with air density overlying the right portion of the cardiac silhouette. A small right apical pneumothorax was also identified.

Differential Diagnosis: Pneumopericardium and pneumomediastinum should be considered.

Diagnosis: Postoperative pneumopericardium with a small right apical pneumothorax.

Discussion: Pneumopericardium is almost always associated with some degree of pericardial fluid that leads to obliteration of the central portion of the diaphragm in the erect position. Pneumopericardium can easily be distinguished from pneumomediastinum with a change in the patient's position and in position of the abnormal gas collection.

Radiographically, gas is noted to outline the mediastinal structures when a pneumomediastinum is present. This is often identified around the thoracic aorta and the pulmonary artery on PA and lateral views. A thin linear lucency is a normal finding along the border of the heart and aortic arch. This Mach band should not be confused with pneumomediastinum. The continuous diaphragm sign arises from air outlining the central portion of the diaphragm. When there is a gas collection between the parietal pleura and the medial portion of the left hemidiaphragm, this outlines the descending aorta in a V-like configuration known as the *V sign of Nacleria.*

CASE 148

History: A 21-year-old pregnant woman presented to the emergency room with acute onset of left pleuritic chest pain. The patient had a history of blunt trauma to the abdomen following a motor vehicle accident 2 years earlier.

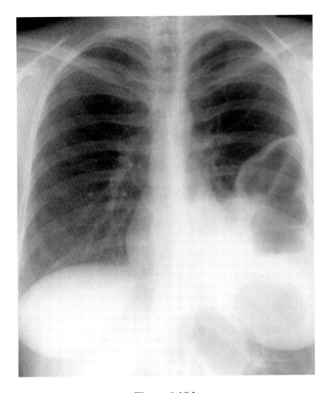

Figure 148A

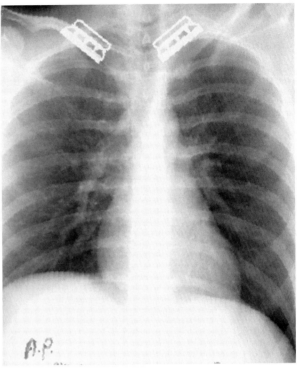

Figure 148B

Findings: A single PA view of the chest demonstrated an air-filled structure in the inferior aspect of the left hemithorax with an air-fluid level within. The left hemidiaphragm was not visualized. An old film on this patient for comparison demonstrated an intact left hemidiaphragm with a well-aerated left lung base.

Differential Diagnosis: Diaphragmatic rupture, elevation of the left hemidiaphragm due to phrenic nerve paralysis, and volume loss from partial lung resection or atelectasis should be considered.

Diagnosis: Diaphragmatic rupture.

Discussion: Diaphragmatic rupture occurs from blunt trauma or from thoracotomy or laparotomy for trauma. It is rarely iatrogenic, and is often associated with hiatal hernia repair or following severe vomiting when it occurs. Potential mechanisms include a sudden increase in the intrathoracic or intraabdominal pressure against a fixed diaphragm, shearing stress on a stretched diaphragm, and avulsion of the diaphragm from its attachment points.

Rupture is often left sided because of the buffer action of the liver, the greater strength of the right hemidiaphragm (proven on cadaver studies), and the underdiagnosis of right-sided injuries. The posterolateral diaphragmatic surface is the weakest along the embryonic fusion lines.

Radiographic results are usually normal or nonspecific, including hemothorax, pneumothorax, and apparent elevation of the hemidiaphragm. Diagnostic signs include a herniated stomach or small bowel into the chest and the presence of a nasogastric tube above the level of the diaphragm. Irregularity of the diaphragmatic contour, lack of visualization of the diaphragm, and elevation of the hemidiaphragm without atelectasis are suggestive radiographic findings. Persistent basilar opacity mimicking atelectasis or subdiaphragmatic mass, and contralateral mediastinal shift without associated large pleural effusion or pneumothorax also suggest diaphragmatic rupture.

CASE 149

History: A 71-year-old man presented with a history of gastroesophageal reflux disease, dysphagia, and regurgitation of food.

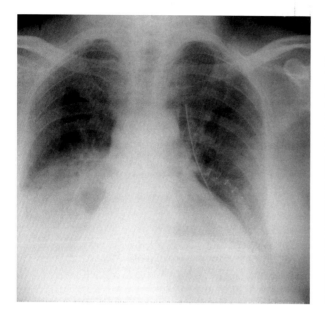

Figure 149A

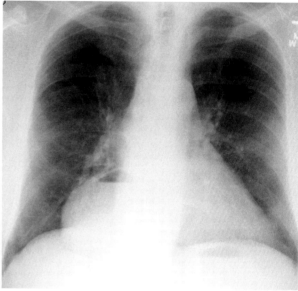

Figure 149B

Findings: A portable frontal view of the chest demonstrated a large soft tissue mass that projected over the right cardiac silhouette and right cardiophrenic angle. This mass demonstrated an air-fluid level within it. The follow-up frontal portable chest film demonstrated recent postoperative changes with a right pleural effusion and left thoracostomy tube with small residual left pneumothorax. A region of residual lucency was again noted overlying the right medial lung base.

Differential Diagnosis: Congenital cyst of the distal esophagus, diverticulum formation secondary to distal esophageal obstruction, and large hiatal hernia should be considered.

Diagnosis: Large epiphrenic diverticulum secondary to achalasia.

Discussion: Congenital esophageal cysts are round, cystlike structures to the right of midline just above the diaphragm. An air-fluid level is usually present. Barium studies are diagnostic. A large hiatal hernia is also represented radiographically as a retrocardiac mass. Although these two entities would be plausible given the radiographic findings, the etiology in this case proved to be epiphrenic diverticulum formation from achalasia.

Achalasia is usually radiographically apparent as a shadow projecting to the right side of the mediastinum. Because it is posterior to the heart, there is no silhouette sign with the heart. There may be anterior deviation of the trachea. Food with an air-fluid level may be noted in the esophagus. Barium studies are diagnostic, but CT also can be confirmatory.

The symptoms of achalasia include dysphagia and chronic cough. Patients may have recurrent pneumonia from aspiration. Some patients may present with stridor.

CASE 150

History: A 73-year-old man with a history of coronary artery disease had undergone coronary artery bypass grafting. He also had a history of gastroesophageal reflux disease, and presented to the pulmonary clinic with the complaint of chronic cough.

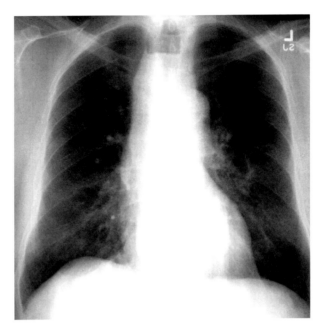

Figure 150

Findings: A PA radiographic view of the chest suggested esophageal dilatation with an air-fluid level overlying the superior mediastinum.

Differential Diagnosis: Stenosis/partial obstruction of the distal esophagus from reflux esophagitis, neoplasm of the distal esophagus or gastric cardia, primary achalasia, scleroderma, and infection with Chagas' disease should be considered.

Diagnosis: Primary achalasia.

Discussion: Of all the entities in the differential diagnosis, achalasia causes the highest degree of esophageal dilatation. It is usually radiographically apparent as a shadow projecting to the right side of the mediastinum. Because it is posterior to the heart, there is no silhouette sign with the heart. There may be anterior deviation of the trachea. Food with an air-fluid level may be noted in the esophagus. Barium studies are diagnostic, but CT also can be confirmatory.

The symptoms of achalasia include dysphagia and chronic cough. Patients may have recurrent pneumonia from aspiration. Some patients may present with stridor. The differentiation between achalasia and scleroderma (progressive systemic sclerosis) is easily made. In contrast to achalasia, there is usually no air-fluid level associated with scleroderma, and the stomach is usually filled with gas. The classic scleroderma lung changes of interstitial fibrosis in the lower lungs also aid in the distinction.

SUGGESTED READING

Adler DG, Romero Y. Primary esophageal motility disorders. *Mayo Clin Proc* 2001;76:195–200.

Bejvan SM, Godwin JD. Pneumomediastinum: old signs and new signs. *AJR Am J Roentgenol* 1996;166:1041–1048.

Baumann MH, Strange C, Heffner JE, et al. Management of spontaneous pneumothorax : an American College of Chest Physicians Delphi Consensus Statement. *Chest* 2001;119:590–602.

Chan L. Medial pneumothorax: a radiographic sign that should not be overlooked on the supine view. *Am J Emerg Med* 1999;17:431–432.

Dunaway PM, Wong RK. Achalasia. Current treatment options in gastroenterology. 2001;4:89–100.

Hall FM. Radiographic diagnosis of pneumothorax. *Radiology* 1993;188:583.

Kadokura M, Nonaka M, Yamamoto S, et al. Five cases of asymptomatic spontaneous pneumothorax. *Ann Thorac Cardiovasc Surg* 1999; 5:187–190.

Kuhlman JE, Pozniak MA, Collins J, et al. Radiographic and CT findings of blunt chest trauma: aortic injuries and looking beyond them. *Radiographics* 1998;18:1085–1106; discussion 1107–1108; quiz 1.

Miller JA, Ghanekar D. Pneumothoraces secondary to blunt abdominal trauma: aids to plain film radiographic diagnosis and relationship to solid organ injury. *Am Surg* 1996;62:416–420.

Murray JA, Demetriades D, Asensio JA, et al. Occult injuries to the diaphragm: prospective evaluation of laparoscopy in penetrating injuries to the left lower chest. *J Am Coll Surg* 1998;187:626–630.

Okereke UN, Weber BE, Israel RH. Spontaneous pneumomediastinum in an 18-year-old black Sudanese high school student. *J Natl Med Assoc* 1999;91:357–359.

Zylak CM, Standen JR, Barnes GR, et al. Pneumomediastinum revisited. *Radiographics* 2000;20:1043–1057.

SUBJECT INDEX

267

Hypertension
fungus ball and, 138–139
pulmonary, 229
pulmonary embolus and, 126–127
Hypothyroidism, Wegener's
granulomatosis and, 56–57

I

Idiopathic pulmonary fibrosis (IPF),
92–93
Immunosuppressives, for treatment of
Goodpasture's syndrome, 55
Infarction, pulmonary, 128–129, 132–133
Infections
Actinomyces, 23
Aspergillus fumigatus, 177
Candida albicans, 34–35
community-acquired, 21
Enterococcus cloacae, 44–45
Mycobacterium avium intracellulare,
59, 134–135
Mycobacterium tuberculosis, 37, 46–47,
59, 79, 91, 116
Nocardia asteroides, 43
pulmonary alveolar proteinosis and,
104–105
recurrent, 4–5
seasonality, 17
Staphylococcus aureus, 22–23
Streptococcus, 17
Influenza, pneumococcal pneumonia and,
17
Inhalation injuries, *Klebsiella* pneumonia
and, 22–23
Interstitial disease
amiodorone toxicity, 106–107
asbestosis, 96–97
central distribution, 78–90
chronic interstitial pneumonitis,
102–103
with cystic changes, 110–113
desquamative interstitial pneumonia,
94
eosinophilic granuloma, 110–111,
112–113
idiopathic pulmonary fibrosis, 92–93
lupus, 95
lymphangioleiomyomatosis, 114–115
lymphangitic spread of carcinoma,
86–87, 88–89
lymphoma, 90
miliary pattern, 116
peripheral, 91–101
with pleural effusion, 114–115
pulmonary alveolar proteinosis,
104–105
pulmonary edema, 76–77
sarcoidosis, 80–81, 82–83, 84–85
scleroderma, 98–99, 100–101
secondary hyperparathyroidism with
calcinosis, 108–109
silicosis, 78–79
tuberculosis, 91, 116
Interstitial fibrosis, 173
Intrathoracic splenosis, 252–253
IPF. *See* Idiopathic pulmonary fibrosis
Ischemic cardiomyopathy, 14–15
pulmonary infarction and, 132–133

J

Juvenile laryngeal papillomatosis, 193,
194–195

K

Kidney transplantation
pulmonary alveolar proteinosis with
Nocardia infection, 58–59
pulmonary nocardiosis with contiguous
thyroid abscess and, 42–43
Klebsiella pneumonia, 22–23
Klippel-Trenaunay-Weber syndrome
(KTWS), 238

L

LAM. *See* Lymphangioleiomyomatosis
Langerhans cell granulomatosis, 110–111,
112–113
Large cell carcinoma, 165
Laryngeal papillomatosis, 192–193,
194–195
Left lingular collapse, 10
Left lower lobe
carcinoid, 6–7
collapse, 6–7, 8–9
Letterer-Siwe disease, 111
Leukemia
adenovirus and, 20–21
chronic interstitial pneumonitis and,
102–103
Pneumocystis carinii pneumonia and,
30–31
right upper lobe pneumonia and, 18–19
Listeria monocytogenes meningitis, 31
Liver disease, pulmonary hemmorrhage
and, 52
Lobar collapse, 1–11
left lingular, 10
left lower, 6–10
right middle, 4–5
right upper, 2–3
Lobar lavage, for treatment of pulmonary
alveolar proteinosis, 59
Lobar pneumonia, 14–15
Lung abscess, 40–41, 123, 124–125
Lung disease, end-stage, 80–81
Lung lesions, cavitary
adenocarcinoma of the lung, 150–151
aspergilloma, 136–137
fungus ball, 138–139, 140–141
lung abscess, 123, 124–125
lymphangioleiomyomatosis, 122
metastases from squamous cell
carinoma, 144–145
mucormycosis, 142–143
Mycobacterium avium intercellulare
infection, 134–135
non–small cell lung cancer, 146–147
pneumatocele, 120
post traumatic pneumatocele, 121
pulmonary embolus, 126–127
pulmonary infarction, 128–129, 132–133
sarcoidosis with mycetoma, 140–141
septic emboli, 130–131
squamous cell carcinoma of the lung,
148–149
thick-walled, 123–151

thin-walled, 120–122
Lung neoplasms. *See also* Carcinoma
adenocarcinoma, 158–163
aspergillus, 177
bronchioloalveolar cell carcinoma, 164
carcinoid, 166
carcinosarcoma, 167
diffuse ossification from mitral valve
disease, 176
granuloma, 172
hamartoma, 170–171
large cell carcinoma, 165
multiple pulmonary nodules, 175–177
non–small cell carcinoma, 168–169
osteosarcoma metastases, 175
rheumatoid nodule, 173
round atelectasis, 174
small cell carcinoma, 155–157
solitary nodule
central lesions, 154–157
peripheral lesions, 158–163
squamous cell carcinoma, 154
Lung transplantation, for treatment of
lymphangioleiomyomatosis, 115
Lupus, 95
Luteinizing hormone–releasing hormone
agonists, for treatment of
lymphangioleiomyomatosis, 115
Lymphadenopathy, small cell carcinoma
and, 156–157
Lymphangioleiomyomatosis (LAM),
114–115, 122
Lymphoma, 90, 218, 220
angioimmunoblastic lymphadenopathy
(AILD), 224–225
aspergillosis and, 177
B-cell, 211, 228
Burkitt's, 211
calcified treated, 228
Hodgkin's, 218, 220
invasive aspergillosis and, 38–39
key imaging findings, 211
T-cell, 224–225

M

Macrolides, for treatment of
pneumococcal pneumonia, 17
MAI. *See Mycobacterium avium
intracellulare*
Mediastinal disease
aneurysm of the aberrant right
subclavian artery, 236
angioimmunoblastic lymphadenopathy
(AILD), 224–225
B-cell lymphoma, 211
bronchogenic cyst, 221, 230–231
calcified treated lymphoma, 228
cystic anterior mediastinal lesions,
204–211
cystic middle mediastinal lesions,
220–222
cystic posterior mediastinal lesions,
230–238
enlarged hemiazygous vein, 238
esophageal duplication cyst, 232–233
fibrosing mediastinitis, 22–227
goiter, 204, 216–217

Renal disease
    diffuse calcinosis from secondary
        hyperparathyroidism from end-
        stage, 108–109
    end-stage, 176
Renal failure, Goodpasture's syndrome
    and, 55
Rheumatoid arthritis, rheumatoid nodule
    and, 173
Rheumatoid nodule, 173
Rheumatoid pneumoconiosis, 173
Right middle lobe, collapse, 4–5
Right middle lobe syndrome (RMLS), 4–5
Right upper lobe
    adenovirus, 20–21
    collapse, 2–3
    pneumonia, 18–19, 20–21

S
Saline lavage, for treatment of alveolar
    proteinosis, 61
Sarcoidosis, 80–81, 82–83, 84–85
    with mycetoma, 140–141
    stage III, 82–83
    stage IV, 80–81
Schwannoma, 242–243
    key imaging findings, 243
Scleroderma, 98–99, 100–101
    pulmonary manifestations, 99
SCUBA diving with bronchial atresia,
    186–187
Septic emboli, 130–131
Silicosis, 78–79
Small cell carcinoma, 155–157
    metastases, 223
Smoking, 2–3, 4–5
    adenocarcinoma and, 158–159, 160–161
    bronchioalveolar cell carcinoma and,
        70–71
    carcinoid and, 166
    centrilobular emphysema and, 182–183
    eosinophilic granuloma and, 112–113
    fungal pneumonia and, 34–35
    invasive squamous cell carcinoma and,
        206–207
    large cell carcinoma and, 165
    lung abscess and, 123, 124–125
    metastatic non–small cell carcinoma of
        the lung and, 219

metastatic small cell carcinoma and, 223
Mycobacterium avium intracellulare
    and, 134–135
non–small cell carcinoma and, 146–147
panlobular emphysema secondary to
    α₁-antitrypsin deficiency, 184–185
pulmonary infarction secondary to
    thromboembolic disease and,
    128–129
rheumatoid nodule and, 173
round atelectasis and, 174
silicosis and, 78–79
small cell carcinoma and, 156–157
squamous cell carcinoma and, 148–149,
    154
thymic cyst and, 205
undifferentiated small cell carcinoma
    and, 155
Splenosis, intrathoracic, 252–253
Squamous cell carcinoma, 154
    of the esophagus, 248
    invasive, 206–207
    of the lung, 148–149
    metastases, 144–145, 250
    Pneumocystis carinii pneumonia and,
        30–31
    tracheoesophageal fistula and, 191
S sign of Golden, 3
Staphylococcus aureus, 22–23
Steroids
    for amiodarone pulmonary toxicity, 107
    for treatment of Goodpasture's
        syndrome, 55
Streptococcus pneumoniae, 17
Sulbactam, for treatment of
    pneumococcal pneumonia, 17
Sulfonamides, hypersensitivity
    pneumonia and, 53
Superior vena cava (SVC) syndrome,
    156–157
SVC. *See* Superior vena cava syndrome
Sympathetic ganglia tumors, 235

T
Tamoxifen, for treatment of
    lymphangioleiomyomatosis, 115
Tension pneumothorax, 258–259
Teratoma, 208–209
    key imaging findings, 209

Thymic cyst, 205
Thymoma, 212–213, 214–215
    key imaging findings, 213
    metastases, 254
    myasthenia gravis and, 215
Thyroid goiter, 204, 217
Tobacco use. *See* Smoking
Tracheoesophageal fistula, 191
Traction bronchiectasis, 96–97
Transplantation
    bone marrow, 44–45, 102–103, 177
    kidney, 42–43, 58–59
    lung, 115
Trauma, 121
Tricuspid endocarditis, septic emboli and,
    130–131
Trimethoprim/sulfamethoxazole
    as prophylaxis for *Pneumocystis carinii*
        pneumonia, 33
Tuberculosis, 37, 46–47, 59, 79, 91, 116
Tuberculous pneumonia, 46–47
Tumors
    carcinoid, 6–7
    paraganglionic, 235
    primitive neuroectodermal, 239
    sympathetic ganglia, 235

U
Usual interstitial pneumonia (UIP), 93

V
Vascular disease, pulmonary infarction
    secondary to thromboembolic
    disease and, 128–129
VATER complex, 191
Ventricular septal defect (VSD)
    pulmonary hypertension and, 229

W
Wegener's granulomatosis, 56–57
White blood cell counts, pneumococcal
    pneumonia and, 17

Z
Zenker's diverticulum
    aspiration pneumonia and, 27
    symptoms, 27